CLINICAL ECOLOGY

A study of how the environment promotes disease or ill health in individuals, and advice on the methods of diagnosis and management of ecological illness.

CLINICAL ECOLOGY

A Therapeutic Approach to Understanding and Treating Food and Chemical Sensitivities

by

G. T. Lewith and J. N. Kenyon

THORSONS PUBLISHERS LIMITED
Wellingborough, Northamptonshire

First published in 1985

British Library Cataloguing in Publication Data

Lewith, G. T.
  Clinical ecology.
  1. Environmentally induced diseases
  I. Title   II. Kenyon, Julian N.
  616.07'1   RB152

ISBN 0-7225-1102-7

Printed and bound in Great Britain

Contents

Introduction

This book is designed to inform the reader how, and to what extent, environmental factors affect our health and in some cases promote disease. Such illness and its treatment is often thought of as 'food sensitivity' or 'allergy'. We feel that the term 'clinical ecology' is more appropriate because it implies a broader view than solely using diets to solve problems. In effect, clinical ecology is the study of how the environment promotes disease or ill health in individuals. Furthermore, it attempts to provide a framework for treating the individual and giving him a system for becoming and remaining healthy. General advice is all very well — we know we shouldn't smoke or become overweight; however, advice tailored to a particular individual's need or a specific problem is of more direct and immediate value.

Many useful books in this field contain dietary lists and detailed instructions that will allow the reader to define his or her food and/or chemical sensitivities. We have chosen not to add to this readily available information, but instead to discuss underlying controversies, conflicts and strengths of both clinical ecology and conventional medicine. By adopting this attitude we hope we have provided the reader with an objective but eclectic approach to this subject.

We both practise clinical ecology and were the first doctors to teach clinical ecology in this country. We believe that in time this therapeutic approach will be used widely, to the enormous benefit of many who currently suffer intractable ill health. Clinical ecology is not, however, a panacea for all ills. It must be assessed and evaluated along with all the other alternative therapies so that it can eventually become established within the framework of normal medical practice.

G. T. Lewith, MA, MRCP, MRCGP
J. N. Kenyon, MD, MB, Ch.B.
The Centre for the Study of Alternative Therapies, 1984

1. What is Allergy?

Over the last decade allergy has been a growth area of medical research. It is therefore important for us to explore what the conventional doctor understands as an allergic phenomenon and to see how this correlates with some of the important concepts in clinical ecology, specifically with respect to food allergy. The science of immunology, the study of the biochemical and physiological mechanisms of allergy, has opened many new doors within medical science and has given us a far more concise understanding of how the body's natural defence mechanism can overcome simple bacterial infection such as acute tonsillitis. One of the major areas studied within immunology is the function or malfunction of the immune system in cancer. All of us regularly produce cancerous cells, but a particular type of white blood cell 'scans' the body and identifies such dangerous incidences. The cancerous cells are then destroyed by the body's 'immune surveillance system', or overt cancer develops if this system breaks down. This type of rigorous and highly sophisticated internal health check is part of our natural physiology. Under normal conditions the body is therefore able to identify normal and abnormal tissue with great accuracy; normal tissue is often thought of as 'self' and abnormal tissue as 'non-self'.

The immune system
The immune system has two main weapons. Initially it produces chemicals directed at the harmful organisms which produce potentially toxic substances that come into contact with the body.

For instance, if a bacteria releases a toxin (an antigen), then the body produces an antitoxin. These antitoxins are called antibodies and are manufactured by a particular type of white blood cell called a B lymphocyte. If we suffer from a localized infection such as a boil, pus is produced. Pus results from a combination of the invading bacteria and various types of white blood cell which eat up the debris produced by immobilizing and killing the bacteria with antibodies. Its second weapon is by means of cell-mediated immunity. The white blood cells responsible for cell-mediated immunity are called T lymphocytes, and phagocytes are responsible for removing and dispersing the detritus. T-cell activity is affected by stress, which may provide an explanation for the observation that stress predisposes to cancer. These two mechanisms, the production of antibodies and cell-mediated immunity, form the basis of our immune or defence system against both internal disease such as cancer and external insults such as infections.

The antibodies produced by B lymphocytes are called immunoglobulins. These are proteins and their detailed chemical structure is designed to bind specifically to the chemical or bacteria defined as harmful (non-self). Under normal circumstances the body is able to recognize its own healthy constituents and consequently (except in some disease states) does not make immunoglobulins or antibodies which destroy its own structures. The antibodies it does make are specifically designed to destroy particular chemicals; for instance, the surface chemicals on a virus will trigger B lymphocytes to produce antibodies against them. The antibodies produced will bind to the viral chemicals very tightly, rather like a lock and key. This alerts other white blood cells so that the invading virus is ingested and destroyed. Once a B cell has produced the specific antibody for a particular virus this 'immune memory' remains, thus providing the theoretical basis for techniques like immunization. A small dose of smallpox protects the body via its immune memory system from the onslaught of the full-blown disease.

Immunoglobulins
Immunoglobulins fall into four main categories, immunoglobulin E, A, G and M, all of which are of similar chemical constitution. Immunoglobulin E binds to cells (mast cells) in the body that contain many chemicals like histamine; the release of histamine into the

skin results in a nettle rash or hives. If an antigen binds specifically to an immunoglobulin E molecule then the mast cell is triggered to release histamine. This results in an acute reaction, often an itchy rash or a sudden wheezy attack. Such reactions are swift, predictable and usually easy to isolate. The foods that trigger this response are often single and eaten irregularly — such as shrimps and strawberries. Consequently this type of food allergy is easy to understand and explain within the context of modern immunology. Immunoglobulin A is produced by the lymphocytes in the gut and is directed mainly at substances in contact with the gut. Immunoglobulin G and M are both found in the blood and are mainly responsible for controlling infectious diseases and acute inflammation within the body.

The mechanism of food allergy

Coeliac disease is not an uncommon condition; it is caused by a reaction to gluten, which is one of the most important protein constituents of grains such as wheat, oats, rye and barley. If a patient is sensitive or allergic to wheat, then continual exposure to this food results in serious but usually reversible damage to the lining of the intestine. This in turn compromises the intestine's normal function and results in its inability to absorb and digest food properly. If the disease was purely 'allergic', one would expect alterations in immunoglobulin A within the gut, and perhaps immunoglobulin A antibodies to the chemical constituents of gluten. However, such reactions do not occur. In spite of this, coeliac disease responds as if it were an allergic disorder. Various drugs which act to diminish allergic based reactions do alleviate this condition and, furthermore, the complete avoidance of gluten cures the problem. But within our highly researched and well-developed concept of immunology we cannot find a purely immunological explanation for the clinical response that occurs in coeliac disease or gluten sensitivity.

Coeliac disease is an excellent example, as it is a well-recognized problem in the context of both conventional and alternative medicine. It has many associated symptoms, such as mouth ulcers and skin rash. Multiple and ill-defined complaints are often an important part of a clinical picture in patients with so-called food allergies but, in common with coeliac disease, patients with other food allergies don't show consistent obvious changes in the immune system.

You would think that if someone was allergic to wheat or milk then these substances would act as antigens and we would be able to measure, with some sort of accurate immunological test, the resultant antibody production. All currently available blood tests designed to investigate food allergy are known to be notoriously inaccurate and unreliable from the clinical point of view. Yet again and again we are shown experiments which suggest that many food allergies do have some sort of allergic basis; for instance, eczema is often helped with anti-allergic drugs such as sodium cromoglycate or hydrocortisone. Why should these chemicals have an effect if the disease does not have some allergic basis?

Allergy or sensitivity?
It is our feeling that much of the controversy about food allergy has resulted from a misunderstanding of the terms involved. Allergy, according to the immunologist, has become a clear but rather narrow science. If a patient doesn't provide a positive response to a scratch test (a small amount of food is scratched into the skin) or a clear antibody in their blood or intestinal lining to a particular food, then food allergy cannot be the problem, in the immunologist's mind. Yet in a large number of instances, such as coeliac disease, removal of the food results in great improvement for the patient.

The clinical ecologist calls this a food allergy, often to the sound of derision from professors of immunology. Perhaps food sensitivity would be a more sensible terminology, as neither the immunologist nor the clinical ecologist need take offence. We feel that much of the debate that surrounds clinical ecology or food allergy has its roots in the semantics and concepts that surround the word allergy. It seems to mean different things to many people.

However, it is encouraging to realize that food allergy, at least in some instances, does have the beginnings of a scientific basis, and further elucidation of its mechanism should result in a broader and more complete grasp of allergy in general. The mechanisms of sensitivity to chemicals, particularly inhaled chemicals such as gas and petrol fumes, remains an enigma. It is probable that contact with these inhaled substances can result in a wide range of internal diseases such as arthritis and colitis (inflammation of the bowel). We will discuss the diagnosis and treatment of chemical sensitivity in a later chapter, but we can make no realistic attempt to explain these observations within the context of modern immunology.

Auto-immune disease

One of the current trends within conventional medicine is to think a disease is auto-immune. This means that the body's immune system is damaging the body itself, resulting in many serious, progressive and chronic conditions. Certain types of inflammatory arthritis such as rheumatoid arthritis fall within this category.

Conventional medicine seems to perceive rheumatoid arthritis solely as a disease of joints with an accompanying and excellently documented immunological disturbance within the blood and tissues of individual joints. We are also aware that the disease can have many variable effects on almost all the tissues and organs within the body. Conventional medicine seems to have become bogged down in analysing the disease process, while the clinical ecologist is interested in what event precipitated the disease. Perhaps it might be reasonable to suppose that all the immunological changes that the conventional doctor studies, with enormous investment in technology and with great interest, are purely secondary; by overemphasizing such potentially irrelevant detail we might miss the cause. We are not suggesting that just avoiding wheat will 'cure all rheumatoid arthritis'. However, as will be discussed in later chapters, approximately 60 per cent of patients with rheumatoid arthritis will respond to an exacting and careful ecological approach. Consequently we must question the commonly accepted idea of auto-immune disease. All the conventional doctor is really saying is that the disease has an associated immune disturbance. Our experience would suggest that many such immune disturbances are either precipitated or exacerbated by foods and chemicals, and consequently defining a disease as auto-immune has little to do with its cause, but simply tells us about the mechanism in a descriptive and symptomatic manner. It is interesting to consider the observation made repeatedly by clinical ecologists that food or chemical avoidance will often resolve the symptoms of auto-immune conditions.

2. Food Sensitivity

Natural diets

Primitive man lived in a constant and relatively stable environment. Any major changes that did occur were usually the result of natural disasters, such as erupting volcanoes or floods. Initially man probably ate what he could gather, such as berries, nuts, leaves and fruits. As he became more sophisticated he began to develop implements to catch and kill small animals like fish, rodents or birds; having probably started as a herbivore (a vegetarian) he graduated to become an omnivore (a mixed eater), but the majority of his diet would still have been vegetarian. Fire, and the ability to cook foods, would definitely have been of enormous advantage to him. The plants and animals that formed the basis of his diet would have been free of chemical contamination; therefore, although the food may have been of poorer quality and more limited in quantity, in an ecological sense it would have been safe.

Poisons

The poisoning of foods, and pollution of our environment in general, began in man's more recent history. Probably one of the earliest and best documented examples is the way the Romans used lead, which they began to mine early in the development of their empire, using it for plumbing systems and glazing wine containers. Lead is easy to work, malleable, doesn't rust and is therefore ideal for plumbing. Until relatively recently lead plumbing systems were a standard part of many large houses, and in some instances still are! We know from the lead content of the human bones at Roman burial sites that chronic lead poisoning must have been endemic within the population, resulting in symptoms such as intellectual impairment and infertility. Indeed, it has been suggested that chronic lead poisoning was one of the many factors that hastened the fall of the Roman Empire!

More recently tobacco and sugar have been introduced into our society. The effects of smoking are well documented and there are few health problems that have not been attributed to tobacco indulgence in one form or another. Sugar, particularly in its refined form, has only recently received the critical publicity it deserves. It certainly causes serious dental decay and is a significant factor in promoting the overwhelming level of obesity in the Western world. Furthermore, the excessive intake of refined sugar may well be one of the causative factors in diseases such as diabetes, heart attacks and strokes.

Salt (sodium chloride) has been used as a meat preservative for centuries, and in fairly recent history reliable supplies of salt were a much coveted possession. In the past, salt was removed from the meat by soaking before it was cooked, but more recently we have begun to add salt to our food in excessive quantities. We probably all consume three or four times more salt than we need. It would seem that in some instances a high salt intake aggravates diseases of the heart and circulation of the blood; the mechanism for this may be through a direct effect on blood-pressure. There is some evidence to suggest that high salt intake causes high blood-pressure (hypertension) and that decreasing dietary salt help to control this problem.

Overall, more than 7,000 individual food items are now in use; many are artificial colourings and chemical additives. Many more are mixed into prepacked and deep-frozen foods that seem to form such a large part of our modern diet. Anyone interested in observing the junk food that is widely available should stand at their local supermarket check-out for an hour or two and watch what people buy. Artificial colouring and preservatives are in regular use to make food look more attractive and increase its shelf life.

Chemical and industrial pollution is also very much on the increase. Although in some areas we are improving our environment, other problems such as acid rain are emerging as

forceful and destructive influences in Europe's ecology. The use of
insecticides, fertilizers and preservatives may be insidiously inflicting
enormous environmental chaos, the full extent of which will
probably only become apparent after it's too late.

Can man cope?

Man's habitat and habits have evolved slowly and painfully over
many millions of years. He has been able to adapt to his
environment within the context of slow change interspersed with
the odd natural or man-made disaster. However, the rate of change
has accelerated out of all proportion, and consequently we feel
that the incidence of ecological disease has also increased in parallel.
Doctors often argue about definition of particular diseases and their
incidence. For instance, the Victorian physician did not use the term
'heart attack' as a diagnosis; any chest pain arising from the heart
was called angina pectoris. We now differentiate between heart
muscle cramp (angina pectoris) and heart muscle damage (a heart
attack). One could argue that the incidence of heart attacks has
really remained constant, and it's just the diagnostic labels that
have changed. We feel strongly that such assumptions do not apply
to ecological illness. We believe the incidence has increased in real
terms and in direct proportion to the extent of environmental
pollution both in foods and from industrial chemicals of various
types.

General advice

Ecology, naturopathy, allopathy and simple common sense are all
giving us the same message. We are polluting our environment
and this is resulting in an increased incidence of disease, primarily
chronic disease. Man is simply not able to adapt to these
environmental changes without some detriment. Not all of us will
suffer symptoms; it's just a small but increasing minority who seem
to over-react while the rest of us are able to cope (at least on the
surface) quite well. However, it is possible that many of our chronic
diseases might be exacerbated by the swift rate of environmental
change occurring around us. As a general principle, both the
conventional doctor and the clinical ecologist would agree that
disease prevention is a better rule to follow than either palliative
or curative measures after the disease has become apparent.

Another general principle that emerges from ecology is that the burden of keeping well or being healthy is shifted from the doctor, or the prescribed medication, to the patient. If someone has migraine due to a milk and beef sensitivity then once the diagnosis has been made the burden of treatment is no longer the doctor's job. The patient must take responsibility for his own actions and the consequent symptoms of abuse. This represents a powerful tool within the general framework of demedicalizing illness. Many responsible general practitioners are continually seeking solutions which make patients less 'doctor dependent'. In a large number of instances ecology is an approach that fulfils this need. In spite of the apparently positive and self-reliant attitudes that are an essential part of the ecological management of disease, many patients seem to choose not to take responsibility for their own problems. We could argue the cause of these attitudes at great length, but it is both important and honest to admit that although the moral and ethical principles of ecology in our opinion are excellent, they are certainly not acceptable to all!

Symptoms

The patient with food or chemical sensitivity often has multiple complaints. A patient is more likely to go to his family doctor with 'legitimate' symptoms such as abdominal pain or headache; he will rarely complain that he feels lousy and tired all the time as presenting symptoms. Headache is a clearly defined complaint and one that fits the paradigms of conventional diagnosis and treatment. If the patient with headache is asked, then he will often volunteer that he has many other vague symptoms, but doesn't feel it's worth bothering the doctor about these. Perhaps he feels (in some cases quite correctly) that many of his other vague symptoms are the product of the severe headaches.

If the initial complaint is vague, such as insomnia, then often the doctor's first instinct may be to suggest the problem is a product of anxiety or nervous tension. In some instances this will be the case, but in others, to put it all down to 'nerves' is a mistake.

Within the doctor-patient relationship the doctor starts off with an enormous advantage — the patient is seeking help and in most instances will listen to and accept the doctor's diagnosis and management. If a particular constellation of symptoms such as lethargy and pain are chronic, then almost invariably the sufferer will become depressed and anxious about his continual state of ill health. Consequently, it is easy for the doctor to convince somebody who is unwell that his problems are all due to his state of mind rather than the converse. While an individual's state of mind is of enormous importance it is sometimes too easy to put symptoms down to anxiety while missing a physical cause for illness.

One of the cardinal rules for the patient who has food or chemical sensitivity is that he almost always presents with vague and ill-defined symptomatology. The doctor frequently cannot explain these symptoms as they don't 'fit' into standard diagnostic criteria. Therefore it is simple to convince both himself and the patient that the symptoms signify anxiety due to marital stress or financial worry. In some instances this may indeed be correct, but we have seen far too many people whose problems respond well to an ecological approach to believe a diagnosis of anxiety without looking a little further than the superficial symptomatology. Taking an ecological history, as well as some other specific diagnostic methods that can be employed, will be discussed in greater detail in the following chapters.

Masked sensitivity

The symptoms that result from ecological illness don't occur immediately after ingesting the food to which the sufferer is sensitive. As previously mentioned, symptoms are multiple and seem to occur randomly. The ecologist calls this a *masked sensitivity*. In other words, the symptoms aren't like a nettle rash or wheezing after ingesting a food to which the patient is allergic; these symptoms occur immediately. In a masked sensitivity a chronic state of ill health develops, such as headache or general malaise. The food to which the patient is sensitive is probably being ingested on many occasions during the day. If the patient is sensitive to milk, then milk in one form or another is perhaps being taken every three or four hours throughout the day. The major problem within clinical ecology is to diagnose the masked sensitivity and subsequently avoid the food.

Richard Mackarness (in *Chemical Victims*) provides a useful analogy for visualizing masked sensitivity. He suggests that the body is rather like a barrel. Usually we can cope with all normal foods and chemicals with which we are in regular contact. These physical stresses can be visualized as water filling the barrel. In other words, most of us are healthy and can cope with most of the stresses (water) to which we are exposed. If we can't cope with these environmental stresses then the barrel overflows and symptoms result.

This analogy has a number of important implications which we would like to look at in more detail. Mackarness's original concept of stresses on the body was limited to foods and chemicals. In our experience environmental stress is an all-embracing concept and must include much more. A child may have a number of food sensitivities, resulting in the symptom of eczema. For most of the year the eczema may be mild and relatively quiescent, it may flare during the winter (climatic stress) or it might worsen when the child changes schools (emotional stress). Consequently, the events causing the barrel to overflow are multiple and, in our experience, include psychological as well as physical stresses.

Western medicine conceives of the disease as the primary event. The ecologist believes that food or chemical sensitivity is the primary event and the so-called disease (such as eczema) is just the body's response to stress. This idea will be discussed in some detail in a later chapter, but it is important to realize that the symptoms may change while the stresses remain constant. A child with cow's milk sensitivity may start life with abdominal colic and end up with asthma. Although the symptoms may change, the primary cause (milk sensitivity) may remain an important and consistent stressor throughout the child's life.

Another important addition to the simple analogy of water in a barrel is that the 'water' is composed of multiple small stresses. A single symptom such as headache may result from sensitivity to milk, potatoes, tomatoes and eggs. In fact most ecologists recognize that masked sensitivities are almost always multiple and have led to distrust of the observation that 'my headaches are only caused by milk'. In this instance the symptom headache may resolve by excluding milk from the diet, but it may also resolve equally satisfactorily by excluding eggs. The body seems to be able to cope with a considerable degree of stress without breaking down and producing symptoms. The implication of this observation is that not all the foods (or chemicals) to which the patient is sensitive need be avoided. If some of the major stressors can be avoided then the symptoms usually settle and the body will be able to cope with the rest.

The ecologist therefore perceives multiple masked sensitivity as the Central aetiological factor in ecologically based problems. In many instances Western diagnosis is based at a far more symptomatic level, while the ecologist claims to be seeking the causative events for the presenting symptoms.

Hypersensitivity and tolerance

Methods for diagnosing masked sensitivity will be discussed in some detail in later chapters, but if we assume that the diagnosis of masked sensitivity can be made, then a particular pattern of events will follow (see Figure 1).

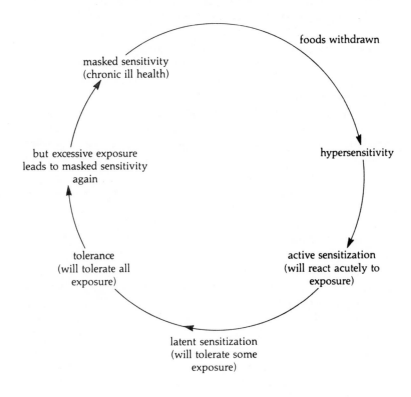

Figure 1:   Diagnosis of masked sensitivity.

Once the masked sensitivity has been defined then the food must be avoided in all its forms. If cow's milk is causing a problem then cow's milk and cow's milk products must be avoided completely (this would include skimmed milk, cheese, whey, butter, etc.). During the first week the patient will often experience cravings for cow's milk in one form or another. He may even have withdrawal symptoms; these symptoms might include a feeling of tension, light-headedness, excessive sweating, diarrhoea and food cravings. The withdrawal should settle after the first week and the initial symptomatic complaint should begin to improve if enough of the masked foods are avoided.

After the first week, but during the first three to five weeks, ingestion of cow's milk will almost always result in acute and unpleasant symptoms. If the patient complains of asthma which seems to settle after a week of cow's milk avoidance, then further ingestion of milk during this time will almost certainly precipitate a severe asthmatic attack. This is called a *hypersensitivity* reaction and will occur (to a greater or lesser extent) in almost all people with masked sensitivity. This hypersensitive stage usually lasts from one week to one month after food avoidance.

After about eight to ten weeks the patient is able to tolerate exposure to the food. Once *tolerance* has begun it can be used therapeutically in the management of food problems. If the patient exposes himself to his sensitive foods too frequently then masked sensitivity will develop again. However, if he exposes himself once every five or seven days then he will usually be able to tolerate the food and masked sensitivity will not recur. This clinical observation underlies the development of rotation diets and allows patients with multiple or major food sensitivities to eat a relatively normal diet providing they plan it in advance. These diets are called rotation diets and simply involve rotating the foods to which the patient is sensitive.

In a few instances tolerance does not develop and patients may remain highly sensitive to particular foods for many years. In other instances the masked sensitivity seems to disappear over a period of a year or two and the patient may be able to go back to eating wheat or milk with regularity, and without the fear of developing further symptoms due to masked sensitivity. However, in general, over-indulgence in a food which has previously caused masked sensitivity is likely to produce further chronic symptomatology.

3. Addiction and Adaption

If you irritate the body regularly but intermittently then it responds with a variety of different symptoms. If the irritation stops then the symptoms often settle quickly, but should the noxious stimulus continue the body tends to adapt and often only a very few minor symptoms result. Eventually, however, the body's adaptive powers are exhausted and severe chronic symptomatology ensues (chronic disease).

Most ecological poisons, at least from the individual sufferer's point of view, are chronic irritants. Hans Selye has described the three stages (acute, chronic and maladaption) as the 'General Adaption Syndrome' (see Figure 2). This principle can be applied to all biological systems exposed to a hazardous environment and the consequent need to adapt to that environment. The conceptual models used to explain clinical ecology correspond very closely to Hans Selye's principle of general adaption.

A simple example of the three stages of general adaption is a chronic physical irritant such as a badly fitting shoe, an example often quoted by one of our colleagues, Dr Patrick Kingsley. Stage one is a sore foot with a blister; if the shoe is discarded the blister will heal. Stage two of the irritation is the formation of hard skin. If the shoe is worn only during part of the day then no pain or other symptom occurs, but the skin hardens. The hard skin will become sore if the irritation is too forceful; consequently even during the most adaptive stage, symptoms can result from excessive irritation. If the shoe continues to irritate the skin then it will break

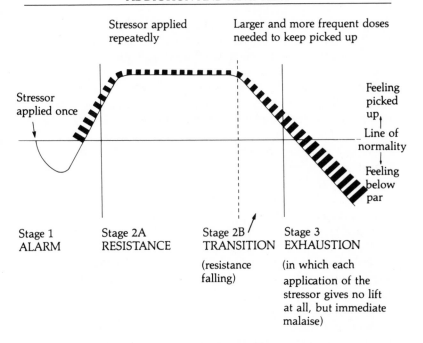

Figure 2: Hans Selye's curve of general adaption.

down; stage three is reached as the body fails to adapt.

Alcohol intake often falls into a similar pattern. Most people dislike alcohol initially. Certainly an excessive intake results in the most unpleasant symptoms such as nausea, vomiting, abdominal pain, vertigo and headache. Prolonged excessive alcohol intake seems to have far less effect. Often the chap who has a 'head for drink' seems to be able to take an enormous amount with few obvious symptoms of drunkenness or hangover. This is the beginning of alcohol addiction or chronic alcoholism. In due course the sufferer finds that he can't start the day without a 'snifter'. He feels ill without alcohol and if he goes too long without a drink unpleasant withdrawal symptoms result, such as headache, nausea and tremor. These can only be solved with the aid of more alcohol; the alcoholic is now well into stage three and unless the addiction and consequent withdrawal can be overcome, death will result.

Addiction and adaption have therefore become intertwined. The body has adapted so completely to the chronic irritant, alcohol, that the individual has become addicted and withdrawal symptoms result if the alcohol is removed. Tobacco addiction is the same; initially everyone hates cigarettes but all too often addiction can result from the chronic abuse of tobacco.

The problems caused by sensitivity to foods or chemicals often follow a similar pattern. A child may find tea distasteful and refuse to drink it but it may be forced on him and eventually he will begin to like it. The adolescent may become addicted to tea and as an adult may begin to develop symptoms such as headache or arthritis. Removal of the irritant stimulus (tea) may resolve the symptoms.

In many instances, however, a single sensitivity such as cow's milk will decrease the body's ability to tolerate other irritants. It will 'drag us down', making us less able to adapt to other potential irritants. People usually don't seek medical help until they become ill. When they experience symptoms severe enough to consult a clinical ecologist, they usually have a chronic and unpleasant illness, almost invariably associated with multiple food sensitivities. In other words, single sensitivities seem to compromise the body to such an extent that multiple problems begin to develop as the body finds it increasingly difficult to adapt to its environment. Furthermore the substances to which the body is sensitive often become the source of an addiction; anyone practising clinical ecology will have come across the 'breadaholic', or the 'milkaholic'.

4. Ecological Disease and its Assessment

People often ask clinical ecologists to define the diseases that are ecological; as if food sensitivity always produces set patterns of symptoms which can be described and placed into some sort of pigeon-hole. The honest answer is that many of the diseases described in the medical textbooks can have an ecological basis.

Differentiated disease
The first factor that we have to consider is, 'What is a disease?'. In conventional medicine a disease is probably no more than a collection of symptoms that 'fit' into a classical diagnosis. The medical textbooks talk about 'the classical history of a duodenal ulcer'; this involves central abdominal pain, often waking the patient at night, and worse between meals. The pain is relieved by food and simple indigestion mixtures. In most doctors' minds the diagnosis of such symptoms is a very simple intellectual exercise but any practising general practitioner will know that such classical symptomatology rarely occurs. All too often the diagnosis is buried and the story is of vague abdominal pain that is difficult to define and certainly doesn't immediately suggest the diagnosis of duodenal ulcer. Therefore classical diagnoses, in our experience, are better suited to textbooks than real life.

Does the diagnosis of a duodenal ulcer tell us anything about the disease? Well, it describes an ulcer or a scarred area in the upper part of the digestive tract (the duodenum); it doesn't tell us anything about the cause of the ulcer or whether a particular patient is predisposed to the development of an ulcer, it simply describes it.

Although the body is a highly complex and ill-understood collection of cells and organ systems, it does seem to have a limited number of ways of reacting to stimuli. Emotional stress often causes us to behave in a particular and predictable manner. It may be that we shout, hide in a corner or go out and get drunk, but for the individual it is often the same predictable behaviour pattern. The cause of the stress can vary from family illness to financial worry, but the individual's reaction often remains the same.

In many ways the body is similar. Arthritis, or painful joints, is an equivalent reaction to that involved in psychological stress. There are two main types of arthritis, active or inflammatory arthritis (rheumatoid arthritis) or chronic degenerative wear-and-tear arthritis (osteo-arthritis). There are a large number of relatively rare small-print arthritic syndromes, but the average GP encounters such rarities very infrequently. It is possible that many different stimuli can cause osteo-arthritis; the search for the elusive cause, and consequent implied cure, may well equate with King Arthur's search for the Holy Grail. It is probable that arthritic change is one of the body's fixed standard reactions or symptomatic patterns

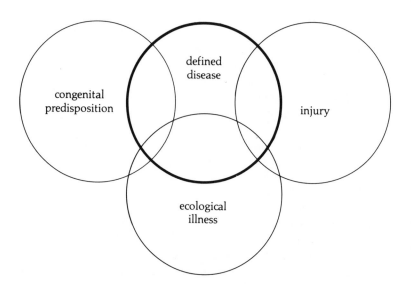

Figure 3:   Diagnosis of differentiated disease.

in response to stress. For some people with osteo-arthritis it seems to run in families (a hereditary predisposition), some have it because of a broken or damaged bone around a joint and some have it for no very obvious reason. Therefore the diagnosis of osteo-arthritis is no more than a symptom pattern or superficial description of a constellation of symptoms. It is not a disease in the complete sense of the word.

In some instances osteo-arthritis does seem to be helped by the use of a food exclusion or ecological approach. This doesn't mean that all osteo-arthritis is an ecological disease; neither does it imply the converse. However, the disease or symptom complex of osteo-arthritis can be alleviated for some patients by appropriate and individually tailored food exclusion. The Venn diagram shown in Figure 3 gives a concise summary of these arguments.

Undifferentiated disease
Undifferentiated disease results in equally difficult problems. If a person develops symptoms that don't 'fit' a conventional diagnosis then the difficulties really begin. GPs are frequently confronted with undifferentiated (in the classical sense), and often undiagnosable, conditions. Hospital specialists rarely see such patients, as most GPs refer patients to a specialist only if they already have some sort of provisional diagnosis. For instance, to whom would somebody with flatulence and malaise be referred? Is this a sufficiently serious problem to warrant a specialist opinion? In most instances, however debilitating these symptoms are for an individual patient, the GP does not refer but soldiers on with a variety of symptomatic remedies.

Because the disease doesn't 'fit', the patient may end up being referred to a psychiatrist. This really represents the doctor's failure as much as the patient's real need. Of course some of us are psychologically disturbed, it's not uncommon; and in a few instances severe distortion of our mental faculties can result in a bizarre collection of symptoms.

Imagine the frustration of a trained professional (a doctor) with a problem patient who doesn't seem to fit into the diagnostic criteria that he learnt at medical school. The doctor's first impulse is not to reject his training, but in a subtle way to blame the patient. He may almost suggest that it's not his (the doctor's) fault that the patient can't be helped, but that it's the patient's fault for being ill. Such frustration is easy to understand and unfortunately all too common. The patient is classed as difficult, depressed, anxious or mad. The doctor uses his powerful status, within the one-to-one consultation, to create a convincing argument. The end result is that the patient often believes that it really is his fault that he is ill, and it's all in the mind! It takes a strong-minded, perceptive and well-informed patient to authoritatively and effectively contradict the medical diagnosis. Most accept the psychiatric label and develop appropriate behaviour patterns in order to cope. We are not for a moment suggesting that all undifferentiated disease is ecological, but we are implying that some of it is. Some is clearly due to emotional trauma, inappropriate behaviour patterns or frank delusion. The Venn diagram in Figure 4 summarizes this argument. Nevertheless all facets of an undifferentiated illness must be considered and it is perhaps wise to ponder on the idea that it is difficult to consider effectively an opinion that you know nothing

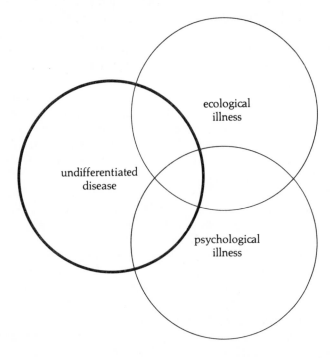

Figure 4:   Diagnosis of undifferentiated disease.

about. Without an understanding of basic quantum physics the atom bomb would not have been possible. How can a doctor seriously consider food sensitivity as the cause of his patient's problems if he knows nothing about clinical ecology?

Perhaps it would be sensible to reconsider the question, 'What is an ecological disease?' The answer still remains that many diseases have an ecological element to them; however, the extent and exact nature of food or chemical sensitivity in particular symptom complexes remains an unknown quantity. We have argued that we believe ecological disease is on the increase — not just the diagnosis of ecological problems, but in real terms. It is almost certain that a small but significant group of people are more prone to ecological problems, while the rest of us can adapt to our environment without too much difficulty. We would therefore suggest that an ecological cause should be considered for almost all medical problems and only rejected if such an approach is obviously inept (as in the case of a fractured leg) or incorrect (for that individual patient).

Assessment
The biggest problem that exists with the alternative therapies is to provide proof, or more exactly 'scientific proof', of their effectiveness. The recent and considerable interest in these areas of medicine has frequently been met with derisory comments such as, 'Show us the evidence, we want proof!'

Those with a good basic scientific training (and we do not consider normal medical training to be a rigorous or enquiring scientific education) would laugh at the claims of 'objectivity', and 'science' made in some of the trials published in reputable journals. The corner-stone of modern scientific drug testing, the double-blind controlled trial (both doctor and patient are unaware of the exact nature of the treatment), is now coming under more concerted attack — both on ethical and pure scientific grounds — than ever before. Such studies are a fairly recent addition to conventional medicine and were unheard of before the 1940s. Most drugs are prescribed by general practitioners and the value of double-blind controlled trials in the context of general practice is open to much confusion and doubt. We are not suggesting that such trials are a valueless method of assessing treatment, but rather that they should be interpreted with caution and not be represented as the final arbiter concerning the value of a particular therapy in specific conditions.

The use of a food exclusion diet as a treatment is difficult to test in this manner. The patient and doctor must know, at least initially, exactly what is happening and what the therapy entails. Therefore the use of a blind study model is inappropriate. (Single blind means that the patient doesn't know whether he is receiving a real or pretend treatment and double blind means that both the doctor and the patient are in the dark about the exact nature of the treatment.) The second problem is compliance. It's all very well asking fifty people with headaches to avoid milk, but will they all do that in a reliable and exacting manner? Will everyone understand that whey is a milk product which is contained in many margarines? Therefore properly conducted studies using food exclusion are difficult to execute and may be difficult to interpret.

One way round these problems is to use an anti-allergic drug. One chemical that has been frequently quoted and tested in this context is sodium cromoglycate (trade name Nalcrom). This acts on mast cells to stabilize the cell membrane and therefore if an antigen hits the immunoglobulin E fixed to the surface of the mast cell, the cell is less likely to release chemicals like histamine. The drug has been used with great effect in asthma; in its inhaled form is called Intal.

If oral sodium cromoglycate alleviates symptoms it seems that food allergy is mediated through the immune response. We would argue that this may not be the case in all instances. Nevertheless, such an approach does have some value and may guide us in identifying patients who have food allergies. In some instances oral sodium cromoglycate is of value, but above all else its use fits the concept of a double-blind controlled study and so is easier (and more acceptable) to assess within the paradigms of conventional medicine.

5. What Diseases Respond to an Ecological Approach?

Ecological (food and chemical sensitivity) disease is more likely to develop in people who have some constitutional predisposition; for instance, food allergies often run in families. Specific common foods such as cow's milk have been implicated in many allergic disorders — from those recognized and acceptable in conventional medicine, such as enzyme deficiencies in the gastro-intestinal tract (and consequent diarrhoea), to those which are less acceptable, such as headaches. Therefore the same stimulus may produce different symptoms in a number of individuals.

IN CHILDHOOD

Food sensitivity usually begins early in life with a few specific symptom patterns. Probably the most important eating habits are established in the first few months of life and this is when most damage can be done to the child's digestive system. It was common for babies to be supplemented with sugar-water or dilute cow's milk-based feeds from a very early age, although the practice is increasingly uncommon. It seems that a small baby's digestive system is not prepared for foods other than breast milk, which is rich in the mother's immunoglobulins to protect the child against external infections. If a child has an allergic predisposition, then the inclusion of any non-breast-milk feeds in the first few weeks of life can begin a cycle of food sensitivity that may be impossible to control except by appropriate food exclusion.

Infantile colic

This is common and often identified by the euphemism 'three month colic'. Almost invariably the cause is, in our experience, sensitivity to cow's milk or cow's milk products. If the baby is being fed on an artificial preparation, then sometimes changing the feed may settle the child. Each commercially available product has the food prepared in a specific manner with a wide range of 'balanced' additives. In some instances just a small decrease in the amount of cow's milk or a slight change in the added constituents can result in significant symptomatic improvement. In other babies symptoms will not settle unless the method of feeding is changed (to breast milk) or symptomatic anti-spasmodic remedies are given.

People who have borderline sensitivities may, at any stage in their lives, effectively manage such symptoms by minor changes in the preparation of their food: for instance, fried eggs may always result in indigestion, but boiled or poached eggs could be fine; a slice of bread may produce symptoms whereas toast may cause no problem. The reasons for this are unclear.

Usually childhood colic is treated by a health visitor or a general practitioner with little or no knowledge of clinical ecology. The baby often remains unwell, with bouts of severe colic after the evening feed associated with foul-smelling and/or green stools. When the child is about three or four months old, the colic begins to settle, and other foods are being introduced so the baby is no longer specifically reacting to cow's milk. In a few, very sensitive, children symptoms of colic may occur even when the child is being breast fed. In some cases it may be necessary for the mother to avoid cow's milk and cow's milk products in order to allow the child to settle. It is unclear as to why this reaction should occur. It's probably not the cow's milk itself, but it may be the mother's antibodies to cow's milk that are secreted in her breast milk. This implies the potential for developing cow's milk sensitivity is strongly bound to the mother's allergic propensity; she is usually cow's milk sensitive and that's why cow's milk antibodies are produced in her milk. It is often easy for the mother to experiment. Any breast-feeding mother will know that if she drinks alcohol the baby will sleep, or if she eats grapes the baby will have loose stools. The same rule can be applied to colic, and in many instances the mother should be able to define the food or foods that diminish the symptoms on abstinence and generate them on reintroduction.

Cow's milk

Over the last few decades we have been almost brainwashed into believing that cow's milk is an excellent food, high in calcium and good for bones! Whilst such propaganda may have been true during the war years it is not the case today. Many large animals, such as the horse, cow and giraffe, have enormous, healthy and durable skeletal structures based purely on a vegetarian diet. It seems both irrational and misguided to consider cow's milk as an *essential food* in the context of an otherwise normal Western diet. Cow's milk has never been consumed by the Chinese, yet their calcium balance is as good as in Western countries. Indeed, excessive cow's milk intake is possibly linked with obesity and diseases of the heart and blood vessels. In general a moderate intake of dairy produce is quite safe and probably beneficial for most people. Nevertheless any experienced ecologist will know that cow's-milk food sensitivity is probably the single most important food allergy in children.

Behavioural problems

Sleep disturbance is probably the most common problem exhibited by young children during the first few months of life. All of us naturally have different sleep patterns, some needing more and some less than others. Normality is difficult to ascertain but usually by about six months most children should be sleeping continuously for about ten to twelve hours a night. A significant number of infants with disturbed sleep have been handled badly by their parents; all too often an inexperienced or worried parent may be unwilling to let a child scream and consequently encourages disturbed sleep pattern with emotional rewards. However, a good number of young children with sleep disturbance have food sensitivity causing colic or abdominal pain which acts as the trigger for recurrent and persistent wakefulness.

Hyperactivity is an extreme form of sleep disturbance. Many parents go to their general practitioner suggesting that their child is hyperactive because he or she sleeps for perhaps only six or eight hours a night, and having been put to bed at eight or nine in the evening, wakes again at four or five in the morning. This isn't hyperactivity in the real sense of the word; a hyperactive child sleeps for only one or two hours a night.

The late Dr Ben Feingold, an American paediatrician, suggested some years ago (in *Why Your Child is Hyperactive*) that hyperactivity was an ecological problem and proposed that the major causes were the additives and colourings and salicylates used in food. Tartrazine (a red or orange dye) was one of the major chemicals implicated.

Many children on the Finegold diet (additive and colouring free) have noticed an improvement; but unfortunately, as with many all-embracing cures, the Finegold diet only works for some. The underlying principle of Finegold's work is that something within the diet must be causing hyperactivity, but putting all the blame on food additives is clearly too simplistic.

True hyperactivity is often responsive to controlled food exclusion and in our opinion an ecological approach should *always* be considered in hyperactive children. Again we would return to our Venn diagram of defined disease (Figure 3); although an ecological approach is frequently useful in hyperactivity, it can't solve the problem for all hyperactive children.

Constipation and diarrhoea

Any child who has recurrent diarrhoea or constipation must be suspected of having food sensitivities. If the gut is irritated it will often produce excess mucus associated with diarrhoea. The parent will frequently comment on the mucous appearance of the child's stools, but will usually be ignored. There's often little to find on detailed investigation, but nevertheless food sensitivity should be suspected.

An enzyme called lactase is produced by the gut, and lactase digests milk. Some Negro and Oriental children have a congenital lack of this enzyme, which means that if they drink milk the milk won't be digested and diarrhoea will result. Lactase deficiency may be an isolated problem, or it may be found in association with other food allergies. The treatment is complete avoidance of milk and dairy products.

In older children, constipation is a more common complaint. Certainly those of Victorian parentage may remember an overwhelming obsession with regular bowel activity. Particularly with our current excessive intake of highly refined foods, it is not uncommon to find children who need repeated encouragement in order to produce regular bowel movements. Although it is important to remember that abnormal bowel habit may result from a variety of behavioural problems in children, a food allergy must not be overlooked. Again cow's milk as well as general dietary advice (more bulk and less refined food) are good lines of attack.

Ear, nose and throat problems

The ears, nose and throat are common target areas for the symptoms of food allergy, particularly in children. Almost any chronic, upper respiratory tract problem in a child might be due to food allergy and this approach must always be considered. As with most other allergies in children, cow's milk is the most common allergen, although wheat and other grains may be responsible for the symptoms.

A well-known general practitioner, Dr John Fry, describes the *chronic catarrhal child*. These three words convey an image of the youngster with a permanently snotty nose who is continually getting colds. There seems to be no good explanation within conventional medicine as to why such a child should be so affected. Acute exacerbations of these symptoms often occur during the winter months, precipitating a visit to the doctor and the all too frequent prescription for antibiotics. In the summer the symptoms are often more settled. The normal history of such children is that they usually have some minor surgical procedure such as removal of the tonsils or adenoids and then grow out of their symptoms. In fact the careful observer will note that a quiescent period may occur after such interventions but further symptoms such as headache, asthma, eczema, or unexplained abdominal pain usually appear at a later date. As well as chronic nasal symptoms, an acute blocked nose or sneezing may also occur in response to specific foods.

Ear infections are a frequent and particularly painful problem. Occasional acute infections of the middle ear (acute otitis media) are distressing but usually harmless as the child's symptoms resolve quickly and it's almost unheard of for there to be any permanent hearing loss. Occasionally chronic inflammation of the middle ear can result from repeated acute infections and in such situations there is some danger of hearing loss resulting. If such loss occurs it's often temporary, but that in itself can make it difficult for the child at school. In our experience a small but significant group of children with chronic middle-ear problems do have food sensitivities and seem to respond well to food exclusion diets. We have had a number of children who have avoided imminent surgical procedures by the simple expedient of avoiding cow's milk and cow's milk products completely.

Chronic or recurrent *sore throats*, including the diagnosis of tonsillitis, may also be precipitated by foods and/or chemical sensitivities. As with all ear, nose and throat problems the odd acute episodes are almost always genuine infections, but children with chronic problems could have an ecological basis for them. The only way to find out for certain is to place the child on an appropriate food exclusion diet and monitor his or her symptoms. Challenging with the suspected allergen, particularly during the hypersensitive phase, should reproduce the symptom that has been cleared by avoiding the offending food.

Eczema

Eczema is an itchy, scaly rash often occurring on the joint creases behind knees and elbows. It has long been known within conventional medicine that such problems are associated with allergy, thus implying that the vast majority of doctors recognize eczema to be a symptom rather than a disease. It is most common in children, usually occurring after the first year of life, although in some instances it can occur in babies. The stimuli that are known to produce eczema are many. It is often worse during winter, particularly when it's windy and cold, and it can certainly be exacerbated, if not caused, by factors as diverse as man-made fibre, clothing in contact with the skin, emotional stress, or allergy to house dust and/or house dust mite.

A number of carefully controlled studies have been published, assessing the effects of an ecological approach in eczema. One of the doctors at Great Ormond Street Hospital for Sick Children has clearly demonstrated that at least 25 per cent (and in our opinion it's probably larger) of children with eczema benefit from a food exclusion diet. Of those children who do respond to food exclusion the items most commonly implicated are cow's milk, eggs, chicken, artificial colourings and preservatives. A well-constructed study using sodium cromoglycate (Nalcrom) also indicated that eczema is often a food allergy. Sodium cromoglycate is a broad spectrum anti-allergic drug; its possible mechanism in alleviating ecological diseases has been discussed in Chapter 4. Children with eczema were first given sodium cromoglycate, and while receiving the drug the eczema, in about 60 per cent of the children, improved significantly. It returned when the drug was stopped and improved again on its reintroduction.

Within the relatively under-researched realms of this subject such studies are important, particularly if they are as well constructed as those we have quoted. It therefore seems illogical to ignore an ecological approach in eczema. Furthermore it's no use the conventional doctor saying there's no evidence; the studies are available and are certainly worthy of detailed consideration. It is wise to remember that not all eczema is due to a simple food allergy; other ecological factors such as sensitivity to house dust, chemicals (domestic and industrial), or even tap water could be at the root of this symptom.

Asthma

The term 'atopic' is used to describe allergic children, the important triad of atopy being asthma, eczema and hay fever. Asthma is a symptom which affects the breathing tubes (bronchi) in the lungs. These tubes have muscle fibres in their walls and if the muscle becomes irritated it contracts. Normally air can flow through these tubes easily, but if the bronchi are constricted air flow is impeded and wheezing results. The aim of conventional management is to stop the smooth muscle contracting by using bronchodilators or by diminishing the excitability of the bronchial tissue in response to potentially allergenic or dangerous stimuli.

The data on food sensitivity and asthma is less complete than that for eczema, but there is considerable circumstantial evidence that a good proportion of asthmatic children may have some food allergies causing, or at least exacerbating, this problem. If the ecological view is taken in its broadest sense (food and environmental sensitivities) then much can be done for young asthmatics with the diagnostic and treatment methods available within clinical ecology. Certainly ecological advice should be sought before steroid drugs are required to control the symptoms.

Conclusion

We have not attempted to provide an exhaustive list of diseases that can be managed with clinical ecology, but we have pinpointed some major areas of interest by discussing the management of some common diseases. Again we would like to emphasize that we do not consider clinical ecology to be a panacea for all ills, but rather an approach worthy of consideration in many common problems.

IN ADULTS

This section will provide a more complete list of diseases that may be amenable to treatment; those conditions covered in the earlier part of this chapter (childhood diseases) will not be repeated here, since the advice given also applies to adults.

Undifferentiated illness

We have discussed in a very general manner the concept of undifferentiated illness. Undifferentiated illness assumes that a patient has a wide range of symptomatology that does not really 'fit' a single (or multiple) conventional diagnostic category. Some of the common symptoms in undifferentiated illness include:

1 *General malaise,* often worse in the early morning, and associated with difficulty in getting going.
2 *Headache.* This can be anything from a stuffy or vaguely unpleasant and heady feeling to overt migrainous attacks.
3 *Fluctuations in weight.* Sometimes such fluctuations may be eight or ten pounds in any one day, some patients stating that they need to keep at least two or three wardrobes as they don't know what they'll fit into when they awake. Such abrupt weight fluctuations almost invariably indicate a food or chemical sensitivity.
4 *Abdominal distension or discomfort.* Many patients complain of a feeling of distension, which is frequently worse after food. This symptom is not part of any conventional diagnosis and patients with this complaint often present having had a number of investigations, all of which were normal. Excessive flatulence may be associated with a feeling of distension.
5 *Unclear mind.* Sometimes called 'brain fag'. Symptoms such as lack of concentration, forgetfulness, unexplained anxiety or mild depression may be associated with a whole series of vague physical complaints.
6 *Excessive sweating.*
7 *Palpitations* of unknown origin. In some instances palpitations occur because of heart disease, but all too often the patient is told that his heart is healthy and yet he still has symptoms. An ecological cause should be considered.
8 *Arthritic aches and pains,* with no clear diagnosis of arthritis on investigation.
9 *Insomnia* and *excessive fatigue.*

Individually these symptoms don't amount to much, but if many occur at the same time the sufferer's life could become very unpleasant. Masked sensitivity makes it difficult for the conventional doctor to consider a food allergy, as no clear pattern of causal events is obvious. Therefore the diagnosis remains elusive and unless the practitioner understands the underlying concepts of masked allergy, a diagnosis of food sensitivity may be open to ridicule. It's all too easy to dismiss symptoms such as anxiety and depression as the product of long-standing neurosis. In some instances psychological disturbances may be the cause of the symptoms, but in many situations neuroticism is blamed without a thorough search for a physical and consequently more easily remediable cause. It's much easier to change a person's eating habits than it is to change his personality!

Obesity

All too often, as a general practitioner, one hears the cry that, 'I don't eat anything but I still never seem to lose weight.' The average doctor's response to this is that the patient isn't being as honest as he might be about his calorie intake. However, the critical doctor must be aware that not all such patients are pulling the wool over his (and their own) eyes all the time.

Dr Richard Mackarness wrote a book entitled *Eat Fat, Grow Thin* in 1958. His diets were based on avoiding commonly allergenic foods such as wheat and milk. The book was a best-seller and even more impressively the diets really did seem to work. Dr Mackarness suffered from obesity himself during this period of his life and by following his own diet he was able to lose weight, but he was more impressed by the fact that it solved his long-standing tendency towards depressive illness.

Some obesity is due to an inappropriate diet (chips, etc.) and some to pure greed, but a significant proportion of the 'I don't eat anything' brigade do have food sensitivities. Carefully designed exclusion diets can and do help weight reduction for those people and in such instances seem to be more appropriate than a high-fibre or calorie-controlled approach. Obesity, like most other problems, is a complex symptom and should be treated on an individual basis rather than applying the same treatment to all those with superficially similar complaints.

Psychiatric disorders

The very suggestion that much so-called neurotic symptomatology such as *anxiety* and/or *depression* can be an ecological problem seems ridiculous. Richard Mackarness, in *Not All in the Mind*, describes an enormous catalogue of patients with seemingly severe personality disorders and depressive illnesses who have all responded to some food exclusion. However, the enquiring and critical clinician finds it very difficult to accept these observations; it just doesn't fit into the framework of conventional medicine. How can such a simple food like wheat precipitate such mental anguish as to cause an attempted suicide? It would somehow be more understandable if a friend had been crushing a few magic mushrooms into the patient's food, but the staff of life, wheat — never!

It is difficult to assess the claims made by Dr Mackarness in a critical and objective manner, particularly as states of mental disorientation and disturbance are almost impossible to measure objectively. Some circumstantial evidence is available, in that it has been demonstrated within institutions such as prisons that *violent* and *aggressive* behaviour by the inmates increases in direct proportion to the amount of fast carbohydrate or junk food in their diet. Sugar also seems to be an important factor in this regard. Although individual case histories, in the scientific sense, are of limited value in proving an argument, I well remember one of my patients with severe manic depression.

Manic depression is a disease in which bouts of severe, almost suicidal, depression occur, interspersed with manic and very active 'highs'. This particular patient had a relatively mild form of manic depression and was able to continue as a senior nursing officer. However, she was in her mid-forties and things were beginning to get difficult both at home and at work. She certainly didn't believe that an approach using food sensitivity could solve her problems. Nevertheless, I suggested she exclude wheat and yeast from her diet and for the first time in many years she emerged from a severe depression without drugs and became quite normal. Belief on behalf of the patient (and in this case the practitioner) do not seem to be an essential prerequisite for the success of an ecological approach.

Mackarness, as well as others such as Doctors Rowe and Randolph (the American founding fathers of clinical ecology), have claimed that food sensitivity can be the cause of *psychotic illness*.

Psychotic illness describes a severe disorder of the mind which involves lack of insight (the TV as a listening device, the patients hear voices, etc.) often severe paranoia and marked thought disorder. *Schizophrenia* is considered to be a psychotic illness. In our limited experience such claims are impossible to prove or disprove. First, it is difficult to get such patients to co-operate with dietary exclusion and, secondly, they have often 'learnt' such abnormal and antisocial behaviour patterns that even if the foods which may be causing their behaviour problems are removed, it is almost impossible for them to relate to people normally. Even if the root of their problem is ecological, it often appears to be easier for them to escape into their fantasy and remain mad.

We simply don't know what percentage of psychological or psychiatric disturbance is precipitated by food or chemical sensitivity, but it is obviously not the complete explanation for all such problems.

Diseases of the ear, nose and throat

Our previous discussion of ear, nose and throat diseases has concentrated mainly on childhood complaints and food sensitivity. ENT diseases in adults produce slightly different but equally common symptoms. *Rhinitis* (inflammation and discharge from the membranes of the nose and upper respiratory tract) is a very common symptom. In adults this complaint is usually caused by inhaled sensitivity, and reactions to dust, spores (mould) and inhaled hydrocarbons are at least as important as the foods, while one of the commonest inhaled sensitivities is to tobacco smoke. Even though the inhaled sensitivity may be the primary event causing symptoms, quite frequently food exclusion can alleviate the complaint by reducing the allergic load on the body. Almost invariably food and inhaled sensitivities occur together in the same individual. Therefore the ecologist can approach rhinitis either with a food exclusion, or by desensitization, or by using both approaches.

Chronic recurrent sinusitis or allergic *inflammation of the pharynx* (throat) or *larynx* (voice box) are also likely to be due to a food or, more frequently, a chemical or inhaled sensitivity. Probably the commonest inhaled sensitivity in adults is *hay fever* (inflammation of the upper respiratory tract due to inhaled pollens). This seasonal event can represent appalling misery for those who suffer; sometimes a food exclusion is an appropriate method of reducing the allergic load, but if this doesn't work, desensitization techniques must be used; the desensitization methods are based on the Miller technique, and are only used by clinical ecologists (further discussion of the Miller technique is to be found in Chapter 8). Diseases of the ear, nose and throat, more than any other group of conditions, require a broader ecological approach than just food exclusion, desensitization often being the only way to help the patient.

Neurological conditions

The commonest disease affecting the neurological system is a *stroke.* Strokes occur when the blood supply to the brain is severely disturbed either by a blood clot (thrombus) in one of the major blood vessels to or in the brain, or by a bleed (haemorrhage) from a ruptured artery. These events occur if the integrity of the blood vessel is disturbed, usually by the deposition of fatty tissue (cholesterol) in the arterial wall. Conventional medicine has recognized that environmental factors such as smoking, obesity, a high animal-fat intake and lack of exercise all represent high risk factors for arterial disease. In other words prevention, in terms of the individual's environment, is being recognized as of more fundamental importance than symptomatic measures such as the use of drugs or surgery. The same arguments can be applied to heart attacks (coronary thrombosis), as the causes are similar in that it is almost always the arteries rather than the heart itself where the problems occur.

Headache and migraine

Headache is probably one of the most common symptoms occurring within the community: it seems that about 20 per cent of the population suffer headache in any two week period of their lives. The severity of this complaint can vary enormously, from the mild but easily forgotten pain to a severe migrainous neuralgia that can keep a person in bed for days. It would be ludicrous to claim that all headaches are due to a food or chemical sensitivity. Stress, anxiety and a whole host of other common and potentially remediable trigger factors must be considered before embarking on a dietary approach.

Headache is a term often used interchangeably with *migraine,*

migraine usually signifying a severe headache. While there is some truth in this idea, migraine is really much more than just a headache. It represents an almost perfect example of the breadth of a typical ecological problem. Migraine headaches are associated with symptoms in a wide range of organ systems, which include:

1 The *eyes*. There are often visual disturbances such as flashing lights prior to the headache.

2 *Digestive system*. A feeling of nausea is common during the attack and may be accompanied by repeated vomiting. General abdominal discomfort may also be associated with migraine and in children 'abdominal migraine' has been described — this is a migrainous-like pain occurring in the abdomen rather than presenting with the symptom of headache.

3 *Nervous system*. Sometimes neuralgias or other temporary malfunctions of the central nervous system can occur.

4 *Muscle spasm* particularly in the neck muscles and occasionally associated with spinal pain in the low or middle part of the back.

5 *Anxiety* or feelings of severe depression are frequently associated with severe recurrent migraine; sometimes these mood changes may be produced by the drugs given to treat or prevent the migraine, and sometimes they are caused by the disease itself.

6 *Circulatory disturbances*.

We know that migraine is a disease complex, so it's easy for us to recognize that these symptoms form part of a larger picture. In many other conditions that often have equally widespread symptomatology, these observations seem to have been overlooked, making it simple for conventional doctors to ignore and dismiss widespread symptoms.

We have known for some years that headaches (including migraine) can be triggered by foods containing tyramine, such as cheese, wine and chocolate. These obvious sensitivities are easily isolated, but masked sensitivity is the basis of most headaches caused by foods and chemicals. Studies at the Great Ormond Street Hospital for Sick Children have demonstrated that almost 90 per cent of children with migraine do have food sensitivities, and that their headaches respond to food exclusion; rechallenge with the appropriate foods resulted in repeated headaches. Milk, eggs, chocolate, orange, tea, wheat and artificial colours were the most commonly identified items. However, other studies conducted on a similar basis suggest that wheat, eggs and citrus fruits seem to be the most common triggers for headaches. The case for food sensitivity being an important precipitating factor in many headaches, and particularly in migraine, is strong. The foods responsible will vary from patient to patient and so must be meticulously isolated for each individual.

A few patients with *multiple sclerosis* do seem to have noticed some improvement on appropriate food exclusion, although it's very difficult to assess objectively the effects of any treatment in this relapsing and remitting condition.

Arthritis

Arthritis is a blanket term used to cover everything from inflammation of the joints to the aches and pains one might experience as winter approaches. Arthritis in the real sense of the word means a joint disease, and in most instances pain occurs on movement of the affected joint. There are two main types of arthritis: *osteo-arthritis* and *rheumatoid arthritis.*

Osteo-arthritis is often described as wear-and-tear arthritis, implying that it is a natural degenerative process. In some people a fracture or other accident may damage the joint, precipitating osteo-arthritis at an early age, while in others osteo-arthritis seems to run in families. Information is now emerging which suggests that osteo-arthritis is not simply wear and tear, but may be due to a more complex metabolic disorder involving joint tissue.

Rheumatoid arthritis is an inflammatory joint disease; the joints are attacked by the body's own immune system, a so-called 'auto-immune disease' (see Chapter 1). The active inflammation of rheumatoid arthritis usually burns itself out after some months or years, leaving painful joints or secondary osteo-arthritis. There are many active inflammatory arthritides such as *ankylosing spondylitis, systemic lupus erythematosis* and *dermatomyositis;* all are auto-immune and in many ways are similar to rheumatoid arthritis, both from their natural history and in their response to food avoidance.

There is a growing body of evidence that suggests a large number of patients with both osteo- and rheumatoid arthritis would benefit from food exclusion. Dr Randolph (of Chicago), Dr Mackarness (previously of Basingstoke) and Dr Carroll (of North Carolina) have all reported remarkable success with food exclusion alone. Dr Carroll's published work suggests that 98 per cent of patients with osteo-arthritis and 91 per cent of patients with rheumatoid arthritis feel some benefit from controlled food exclusion. The foods to which patients are commonly sensitive include corn (maize), wheat (and other grains such as rye and oats), cow's milk, tea, coffee, sugar and red meat. Our impression is that Dr Carroll's claims are over-enthusiastic, but nevertheless make the point. A high proportion of patients with arthritis (both osteo- and rheumatoid arthritis) will obtain clear benefit from appropriate food exclusion. The benefit is not simply due to weight loss, but represents a real change in the activity of their arthritis with associated changes in the blood tests. Both the symptoms and blood tests become abnormal again when the patient is challenged with the food to which he is sensitive.

Broad spectrum anti-allergic treatments such as enzyme potentiated desensitization (see Chapter 8) also result in significant improvement in many patients with arthritic conditions. In a few instances it seems that the X-rays begin to change and joints begin to look more normal, although many doctors feel that an ecological approach controls symptoms and stops the condition becoming worse rather than 'curing' anything.

The application of a universal diet for arthritis is, in our opinion, ludicrous. Although certain sensitivities are common, such as cow's milk or wheat, the essence of clinical ecology is that a specific group of foods must be excluded if an individual is to benefit. The food exclusion diet must be based on that individual's needs. Any 'across the board' diet for all arthritics is bound to fail in at least 30-40 per cent of situations; arthritics have a great deal to gain from a dietary approach, but the approach must be tailored to the individual, and based on a critical assessment of his or her response to treatment.

Back pain
Along with headaches, back pain is an almost universal human complaint, affecting 80 per cent of the United Kingdom population at some time in their lives. There are obviously many varied causes of spinal pain, and pain caused by injury or accident cannot possibly be due to a food or chemical sensitivity. Our practice involves the

use of acupuncture and spinal manipulation, two therapies which are frequently very effective in helping sufferers from spinal pain. However, we remain both amazed and impressed that a small but significant number of people who fail to respond to physical treatments do sometimes gain enormous improvement from appropriate food exclusion.

Diseases of the digestive tract

It seems logical that the largest and best researched group of conditions which are known to be food allergies are the diseases of the digestive system, the tissues in closest contact with the food.

Gluten sensitivity (coeliac disease) has been a well-defined food allergy for some years. It was initially recognized by an English doctor, Samuel Gee, at St Bartholomew's Hospital in 1888, but is described more accurately by a Dr Dickie, a Dutch physician, in the 1950s. It seems that the husk of cereals (gluten) damages the gut, so that it fails to absorb other foods properly. Although this has been called an allergy, its immunological mechanism remains largely unidentified. The generalized malabsorption that occurs as a consequence of damage to the intestine is important and seems to be a frequent accompaniment to ecological problems, whether they have produced gastro-intestinal symptoms or not. Gluten sensitivity is a single food allergy; gluten avoidance almost always solves the problem completely and reintroduction of minute amounts of gluten will cause a further relapse. In some instances a picture of coeliac disease is present, but it doesn't seem to respond to gluten avoidance. Dr Asquith from Birmingham has noted that avoidance of soya products often settles these recalcitrant problems. This implies that, although in the classical conventional sense gluten sensitivity is a single food allergy, it may have much more in common with multiple food sensitivities normally found in other ecological diseases.

Indigestion is a symptom that covers a multitude of ills; it can simply be the product of too much food or may signify stomach acid reflux into the oesophagus (*hiatus hernia*) or an *ulcer* in the stomach or duodenum. The cure for over-indulgence is to eat less, hardly a food sensitivity!

In most other instances, food sensitivity is certainly worthy of detailed consideration. Duodenal ulcers are often treated with bland diets which contain lots of milk to soothe the healing skin of the ulcer. I well remember a patient who seemed to be continually developing ulcers and was drinking more and more milk as directed by his specialist. In the fullness of time it became apparent that he was developing his ulcers in response to a milk sensitivity! It has been demonstrated quite clearly that chronic gastritis (inflammation of the stomach) will also respond to food exclusion and therefore there is a good basis for suggesting that many upper gastro-intestinal problems may have an ecological basis. The symptoms of *nausea* and *vomiting* may also be associated with food sensitivities, either as single unexplained symptoms or as part of a broad symptom complex, as in migraine.

Inflammatory bowel disease

Inflammatory bowel diseases are conditions in which the lining of the bowel becomes inflamed and ulcerated. The cause in most instances is said to be auto-immune, which strongly suggests food sensitivity may be a precipitating factor in such problems. There are two main inflammatory bowel diseases, *Crohn's disease* and *ulcerative colitis*.

Crohn's disease tends to be located in the small bowel and ulcerative colitis in the colon, although the two conditions can occur anywhere in the digestive system. They produce slightly different reactions in the bowel wall.

Crohn's disease does respond to food exclusion. Dr Hunter from Cambridge recently reported that approximately 75 per cent of patients with this condition improved on an exclusion diet. The picture with ulcerative colitis is similar, in that a high proportion of patients suffering from this condition will respond to appropriate food exclusion. It is interesting to note that sodium cromoglycate (a broad spectrum anti-allergic drug) has been used to good effect in controlling colitis in approximately 70 per cent of patients. Conventional treatment for inflammatory bowel diseases may involve large doses of potentially dangerous drugs such as steroids. Food exclusion is a harmless treatment, if used responsibly, and must be considered as an option for these complaints.

Irritable bowel syndrome

Irritable bowel syndrome is really a dumping ground for patients with symptoms referred to the bowel but with no obvious conventional diagnosis such as ulcerative colitis. It involves vague

symptoms such as abdominal pain and distension and is said to
have no known cause but frequently occurs in tense and anxious
individuals — this is the conventional doctor's way of blaming the
patient rather than the inadequacy of allopathic diagnosis and
investigation. In our own experience irritable bowel syndrome
almost always improves with food exclusion. Conventional
medicine has little to offer except tranquillizers in various shapes
and sizes; an ecological approach is far safer and more likely to
be effective.

Unexplained abdominal pain
A small but significant group of patients attending the specialist
gastro-enterological clinics present with abdominal pain of
unknown cause; occasionally a diagnosis of irritable bowel or
spastic colon is suggested, but the honest physician may simply
be unable to make a rational assessment of the cause of the pain.
In some instances the diagnosis becomes obvious in time, the pain
preceding other pathological changes which will make the diagnosis
obvious. However, in other cases such pain may remain
unexplained for years. In our experience an ecological approach
is both a worthwhile and frequently fruitful method of
management, food sensitivity being common in such situations
and appropriate food exclusion often resolving the symptoms, to
the satisfaction of both patient and doctor.

Diseases of the heart and circulation
We have already mentioned general environmental factors that
influence the development of arterial disease. Arterial disease is
the central pathology in almost all diseases that involve the
cardiovascular system (heart and circulation). The general and
widely available advice about the development of fatty plaques
(atheroma) within the arteries should be followed. These are:

1 Decrease fat intake, particularly animal fat.
2 Take regular exercise.
3 Learn to develop some relaxation techniques so that you're not
   rushing around all the time.
4 Remain slim.
5 Don't smoke.

Such general ecological advice can be applied to all and is certainly having an enormous effect on the morbidity and mortality of cardiovascular disease in the United States. However, as we have mentioned before, dietary advice designed for the individual is likely to be more specific and has a better chance of success.

Particular problems such as *palpitations* or *angina* (heart muscle cramp) may respond to an exacting ecological approach. I well remember one patient who developed angina every time he drove his car. The superficial explanation would be that the stress of driving resulted in increased demand by the heart for oxygen, and because of the diseased blood vessels the heart didn't receive enough oxygen and so angina or cramp resulted. On testing, this man was sensitive to petrol fumes, with the circulation of the heart apparently being the target organ. In other words, contact with petrol fumes resulted in spasm of the heart's arteries, decreased blood flow and consequent angina. Therefore we consider that an approach using food and chemical sensitivity is of value, even in what at first seems an impossible situation.

Skin diseases
We have already discussed *eczema* and demonstrated the powerful connection that exists between food sensitivity and this condition. It is important to remember that many of the substances in contact with the skin may cause a local allergic reaction such as soreness, and scaly or weeping areas. This *contact dermatitis* is solved simply by avoiding exposure. First look for potential contact allergens and remember that some may display a pattern of masked sensitivity; the contact may be so repeated and chronic (i.e. clothes made from man-made fibres) that isolating the contact allergen may be difficult. If this simple approach fails to produce a result then a more exacting search for foods and chemicals is often both appropriate and rewarding. *Acne* and *chronic urticaria* (chronic skin irritation) are particularly likely to respond to food exclusion. The sensitivities are almost always masked even to foods, but occasionally an immediate worsening may occur after ingestion of particular substances.

Psoriasis does not respond well to an ecological approach.

Diseases of the urinary system
Probably the commonest disease of the urinary tract is *cystitis,*

or inflammation of the bladder. This results in a painful and frequent desire to urinate. Acute attacks are almost always caused by bacteria and resolve adequately with antibiotics. However, those who suffer from repeated acute attacks of cystitis may,in some instances, develop chronic bladder or urinary symptoms. These people do not respond well to antibiotics and often experience great difficulty in finding any solution which will ameliorate their problems. In some instances an *irritable bladder* develops, which can cause severe and intractable pain.

Underlying this type of problem is often a chronic infection with *Candida (thrush)* (see Chapter 11), which is frequently associated with multiple food and/or chemical sensitivity. The conventional treatment of chronic or irritable bladder is not always successful and an ecological approach with appropriate food exclusion is frequently a valuable and worthwhile therapeutic regime. If chronic thrush is the problem it is essential that it should be treated, and this will be discussed in some detail in Chapter 11.

Enuresis (bed-wetting) is not an uncommon problem in young children. It can usually be contained within the family until the child starts to go to school, and at this stage persistent bed-wetting will cause difficulties when he or she wants to spend the night with friends. A food exclusion (often milk) approach can be of enormous value and is successful in many children we have treated with this problem. It is important to bear in mind that bed-wetting may result from an anatomical abnormality in the bladder or elsewhere in the urinary tract; children should be properly investigated before making a diagnosis of 'enuresis, cause unknown'.

Gynaecological problems

An organization called Foresight (Woodhurst, Hydstile, Godalming, Surrey GU8 4AY) has probably done more than anyone to analyse the ecological factors surrounding healthy *labour* and *delivery*. Their literature and advice is sound, and anybody thinking of having a baby would be well advised to read their views on *preconceptual* and *antenatal* care; their approach, although it remains to a certain extent untested, seems likely to produce a safer labour and delivery, with a healthier baby and mother as the end-result.

There are two common gynaecological problems that are amenable to an ecological approach — *dysmenorrhoea* and *premenstrual tension.* Premenstrual tension is often due to a vitamin deficiency (Vitamin B_6) or a trace metal imbalance. Hair analysis for trace elements often demonstrates the underlying cause, although food sensitivity may also precipitate the heavy unpleasant headachey feeling that seems to occur with this condition. As will be discussed in the chapter on hair analysis (see Chapter 10), abnormal levels of trace metals predispose to an ecological problem. Premenstrual tension is rarely due to a simple food sensitivity, and is unlikely to be corrected by food exclusion alone. Dysmenorrhoea is often associated with premenstrual tension and frequently follows the same pattern; trace metal imbalance often underlies a variety of food and chemical sensitivities that settle if treated appropriately. An ecological approach is of value in these conditions, but the therapist must use more than simple food exclusion to obtain good results.

Conclusion
In this chapter we have attempted to discuss a wide range of conditions and suggest which of them might be amenable to an ecological approach. It is impossible for us to cover the whole of medicine in so short a book, but we have tried to give the reader a broad overview of the conditions that we believe can be successfully approached within the techniques available to clinical ecology.

Our practice involves the use of a number of techniques within alternative medicine, clinical ecology being an essential and integral part of this approach. However, we do not believe that clinical ecology is a panacea for all ills, and it would be illogical and slightly alarming should we make such claims. Although we believe that ecology has a great deal to offer and will frequently be the only approach required to solve a problem, we also believe it to be of great value when used in combination with other techniques such as homoeopathy or acupuncture.

The ecologists claim that food and chemical sensitivity represents the causative event in the initiation of particular disease processes (or groups of symptoms). In many instances this may indeed be true, but in other cases it would seem that ecological phenomena are secondary to the insults from infections or chemical poisoning. In other words, food sensitivity can develop in response to other primary stressors.

6. A Patient's View of Ecology

The initial approach of any ecologist will vary according to the techniques he or she favours. Some will advise a five-day fast followed by reintroduction of foods, while others may use intradermal skin testing, electrical methods or one of the other diagnostic techniques mentioned. The majority of ecological problems will respond to simple food, and in some cases chemical, avoidance. In our experience most ecology patients have a number of common questions. They are:

1 How strict do I need to be with my diet; when and how often can I take risks?
2 What are my chances of improving my symptoms, using an ecological approach?
3 How long will it take me to get better?
4 Will I ever be able to eat the foods to which I am sensitive again?
5 Do I need to change my lifestyle?
6 Can I stop my drug therapy?
7 Will my condition relapse?

We will deal with each of these questions in turn so that anybody contemplating an ecological approach will have some idea of the course upon which they are embarking.

How strict do I need to be with my diet?
If you are somebody who reacts markedly to conventional drugs

and/or you know that your reactions to particular foods are prolonged and dramatic, then you need to be scrupulously careful about following your practitioner's instructions on food avoidance. Beware of eating in restaurants or with friends, unless they understand the importance of your diet. It is all too easy to be persuaded to take a forbidden food by an ignorant, but perhaps well-meaning, friend. Make sure you know where your forbidden foods may occur, especially if you are sensitive to a staple food such as wheat, milk, corn or eggs. It is most likely that one of your sensitivities will include one, and in some cases more, of these foods. You may ingest one of these foods inadvertently: for example, you may eat chips which have been fried in fat used for cooking fish in batter; the fat will then contain traces of wheat. If you are wheat sensitive this inadvertent contact may be enough to give you symptoms lasting from a few hours to three or four days. If you are of average sensitivity then occasional inadvertent lapses will not be as serious. In *all* cases, once food sensitivity has been diagnosed, merely cutting down on the offending foods will not do; they must be avoided completely.

When you have avoided a suspect food for approximately six months (for the average patient), then it is possible to eat it occasionally — such as at a dinner party or other similar occasion. The amount eaten isn't as important as the number of times it is taken. If you are going to break your diet, then try and do it at one meal rather than spreading it across a number of meals.

What are my chances of improving, using an ecological approach?
If your illness is one which is likely to respond to an ecological approach, then you have an approximately 60 per cent chance that an ecological approach may help you, either completely or in part. Usually simple avoidance is all that is required. Thankfully, the more complex patients that are discussed elsewhere in this book are a minority. It is important to understand that the sooner an ecological approach is tried for your problem then the more likely it is to succeed. Don't wait until you have run the gamut of conventional drug-based approaches; use an ecological approach as soon as possible. Ecology is best used as a primary care technique rather than a last ditch approach, but unfortunately, in common with many of the other medical alternatives, it tends to be used last. The fact that it works so often in these situations says much for its efficacy.

How long will it take me to get better?

The average patient may expect to experience relief, or in some cases complete alleviation of symptoms, within two weeks. Some problems take longer for an improvement to occur, notably rheumatoid arthritis. A vexed question is whether avoidance of the offending foods enables healing to take place. In many cases this does indeed occur, but it depends to a large extent on how much degenerative disease was present in the first place. For example, an arthritic patient cannot expect his joints suddenly to regenerate. They may well improve so that no pain occurs, but normal mobility may not return.

Many patients, not unreasonably, would define getting better as the stage at which they are able to eat their offending foods without a recurrence of symptoms. This generally happens after approximately two years of avoidance, at which time it is wise to eat the previously sensitive foods on a rotation basis rather than regularly, otherwise the whole cycle will be triggered again.

Some food sensitivities are fixed; this applies most commonly to milk and is usually due to an enzyme deficiency. Some recent research work suggests that patients with multiple sensitivities may have a number of enzyme deficiencies, and this may open up new possibilities for treatment in the future.

Will I ever be able to eat the foods to which I am sensitive again?

The previous section partly answers this question. From a practical point of view it is possible to start a rotation diet some six months after initial food avoidance. If symptoms begin to creep back following the commencement of a rotation diet, then the original foods will have to be eliminated again. As a general rule it is wise not to eat foods to which you have been sensitive on a 'three times daily' basis ever again.

Do I need to change my lifestyle?

Yes, there is considerable evidence to show that many aspects of modern civilized life are unhealthy. The three main areas relevant to ecology patients are the consumption of processed foods, tap water and chemical pollution.

All processed foods, such as tinned and packeted foods (convenience foods), must be avoided. Tap water should be filtered before cooking foods in it or using it to make any sort of drink.

People living in rural areas, or in towns but well away from heavy industrial installations or busy roads, would be well advised to collect rain water from their roofs, using a galvanized iron container. Bottled spring water is an acceptable, if expensive, alternative. Chemical pollution should be minimized by throwing out all spray polishes, deodorizers, window cleaners, etc. Chemical cleaning materials are best replaced by safe cleaning products such as those made by the Shaklee company (see page 84).

Open gas fires or calor-gas heaters should be avoided, as should synthetic materials of all sorts. Food containers should be made of earthenware, glass or hard plastic such as Bakelite. (These latter recommendations are only of major importance to chemically sensitive patients.)

Can I stop my drug therapy?

Many patients trying an ecological approach are on long-term drug therapy of some sort. In some cases, particularly asthmatics and some patients with rheumatoid arthritis, these drugs may be steroids. On no account should any drug be suddenly stopped, and if drug therapy is to be reduced it should be done under medical supervision. This is particularly important for patients on steroids or anti-hypertensives (blood-pressure tablets). Generally speaking, patients who are on long-term drug therapy look for alternative approaches either because the conventional therapy isn't controlling their symptoms adequately or they wish to get off drugs because of fear of long-term side-effects. Whilst this is a laudable aim it should be remembered that in spite of the bad press that modern drug therapy now receives, it does in fact relieve, at least partially, many troublesome symptoms. As a rule of thumb our practice is to see if the patient improves using an ecological approach whilst still taking his or her drug therapy. If improvement occurs, then we slowly reduce drug therapy, with the consent and co-operation of the patient's general practitioner, with the ultimate aim of managing the problem without recourse to drugs. In many cases this is possible; in other more chronic and serious conditions, a reduction in drug dependence, particularly where steroids are concerned, is all that can be achieved.

There is one exception to this rule and that is where the patient is reacting adversely to his or her drug therapy. This can be difficult to recognize clinically and really needs a testing method of some sort in order to diagnose it with any reliability. These patients require a doctor to manage them, as an uninformed approach could be dangerous.

Will my condition relapse?

If the average ecology patient follows the advice set out in this book then relapse will be rare providing long-standing degenerative illness, such as severe arthritis, has not been present before the ecological approach is tried. In this latter group of patients relapses do sometimes occur, usually due to the development of new sensitivities. Their management has been outlined elsewhere in this book, and thankfully these cases are a minority.

Conclusion

Clinical ecology is a simple, safe and often rewarding approach to a wide range of chronic diseases. Most simple ecological problems are not beyond the wit of the man in the street to sort out himself with the help of a practical guide, such as we have tried to provide with this book. We feel that one of the major advantages of this approach is that it puts the onus for an illness-free life on to the patient, and that has to be a healthy view.

7. The Ecology Debate

The idea that illness can be due totally or in part to the food we eat remains a controversial one within conventional medicine. The reasons for this are not easy to find as it is common sense that something we do to ourselves three times daily for most of our lives may be a major determining factor of our health. Perhaps two of the reasons may be the resistance to new ideas by modern scientific medicine and its dominant specialist constitution.

New ideas in medicine
The quantum physicist, Max Planck, said, 'An important scientific innovation rarely makes its way by gradually winning over and converting its opponents. What does happen is that its opponents gradually die out and the growing generation is familiarized with the idea from the beginning.' Orthodox medicine is slow to accept new therapies and quite reasonably expects a good body of evidence to be available before these ideas are accepted. This evidence is gradually accumulating but unfortunately some of it is conflicting and doesn't fit in with current theories of disease causation. Additionally, contrary to the textbooks and philosophers of the scientific method, bad ideas are rarely proved wrong in medicine; they are simply forgotten. The true test of scientific ideas is not its checking mechanisms but a much more objective judge — time. These factors mitigate against critical acceptance of the ideas of ecology by orthodox medicine, with the result that two opposing camps have developed — the ecologists with evermore entrenched

views and orthodox medicine holding similarly entrenched ideas, with neither side being able to look at their own ideas critically.

Specialism

The split into specialist camps is characteristic of the path modern medicine has followed over the past century. There has been, and still is, a strong tendency towards specialization which perhaps explains this polarization. This is probably a reflection of our modern approach to life in that it is fashionable to be a specialist, and 'down-market' to offer a number of approaches. Unfortunately the trend of specialism has been accelerated by our educational system, with its emphasis on a narrowing of subjects studied from an early age. The 'disease of specialism' has even spread to the patient who sees a generalist approach, best represented by general practice, as being second class. Specialism does have its positive aspects, but our point is that we feel that it has gone too far in one direction. It has led to vested interest and, in some cases, tragically inappropriate treatment.

Vested interest in medicine

The modern trend in cardiology for highly technological and expensive coronary care units is a good example of vested interest. Recently a number of studies have looked at the efficacy of coronary care units for the intensive care of patients who have recently had heart attacks. The majority of these studies showed that treatment in such units carried no significant therapeutic advantage to home-based care. One study, however, did show a statistically significant difference in results between the home-based group and the group in the coronary care unit; the patients at home did significantly better than those in hospital! These findings were presented (before publication) to the chief of the coronary care unit concerned but were mistakenly presented the wrong way round (i.e. with the implication that the hospital group did better than those at home). The cardiologist concerned reacted strongly and said that this was the long-awaited vindication of coronary care units. Then the mistake was realized and it was pointed out that the results were the converse. The cardiologist could not be persuaded to change his view of coronary care units.

Specialism encourages a narrow view of illness and engenders a trend to putting diseases into neat diagnostic boxes. The prevailing task of the specialist often appears to be one of semantics, with the initially enthusiastic collusion of the patient in hot pursuit of a name for his ailment. Once the diagnostic label has been handed down, often at enormous expense in terms of diagnostic tests, the patient obtains some short-lived satisfaction. When this runs out then the true quest for a solution begins.

Ecology breaks all the rules by cutting across the artificial boundaries of specialization and also allows the beginnings of an explanation for the increasing number of diseases that don't fit into neat diagnostic boxes. Perhaps an important feature of ecology is that it encourages a novel and more holistic view of illness, but unfortunately ecology itself has developed into a speciality. Perhaps the disease of specialization is endemic to all medicine.

A causally directed view of illness

Modern medicine, in spite of protestations to the contrary, has a predominantly symptomatic approach to illness. For example, arthritis is usually dealt with by pain-killers and anti-inflammatory drugs. There is little attempt to try to determine and then remedy factors which may have caused the inflammation or wear and tear of the joints in the first place. Ecology offers the possibility of a causally directed approach to illness; in other words, it allows causative environmental factors to be identified and then removed with consequent resolution of the problem if the diagnosis is correct. It is curious that there is resistance to this sort of approach within the medical profession. This may have something to do with the constant brainwashing of doctors, particularly general practitioners, by drug companies. As a result approaches concentrating purely on symptom suppression have been given the cloak of academic respectability. The medical management of asthma, for example, has been criticized as a euphemism for symptom suppression, often with steroids. To a certain extent this is true but many asthmatics are also given Intal (sodium cromoglycate), a drug which suppresses allergic reactions. Many doctors would argue that this is a causally directed approach, which to an extent it is. However, if it were possible to identify the factors which caused the allergic reaction in the first place and these were removed, then it would be possible to treat the asthma without drugs at all.

A critical view of the ecological approach

The ecological approach to illness has been taken up with some enthusiasm and some lack of criticism by a few doctors and many patients. The result has been that ecologists tend to see all illness in terms of environmental causes. In practice the ecological approach works well for a wide range of disease, but *a few patients* using this approach have noticed some drawbacks, most commonly that the patient, having been better initially, then relapses. The ecologist then assumes that other hitherto latent sensitivities have now come to the surface, and need to be isolated. For a while this approach seems to work as more and more sensitivities are found with consequent increasing limitations on the sort of life the patient can expect to lead. Eventually it becomes apparent that as soon as one sensitivity has been found another develops. The ecologist, however, remains convinced that environmental causes are primary and the patient is locked into a medical (albeit unconventional) merry-go-round. Perhaps because ecologists have been so beleaguered, they have been unable to ask themselves whether the food and chemical sensitivities are not themselves manifestations of an underlying cause. Our work with the small proportion of severely sensitive patients has led us to believe that many of these problems have underlying causes.

The ecologist cannot be blamed for not looking behind the patient's sensitivities, as even the allergists remain preoccupied with allergy and have not begun to address the question as to why the patient has become allergic in the first place.

Underlying causes of food and chemical sensitivities

Our work with multiple food and chemical sensitivity has led us to look behind these sensitivities in order to devise a manageable treatment programme for many of these patients. The few patients who require this approach are those whose problem has responded initially to an ecological approach and who have been successfully desensitized but unfortunately keep developing new sensitivities. Many such patients, if managed ecologically, lead a more and more limited life and if desensitized may collect enormous numbers of desensitizing solutions, in many cases well over fifty. Because these patients keep developing new sensitivities we have thought that this indicates we are not dealing with the primary problem but treating their sensitivities. Thankfully this group of patients is very small in relation to the total who have problems amenable to an ecological approach, but unfortunately it is a growing minority and so it is of increasing urgency that the limitations of an exclusively ecological approach are recognized. However, many of our insights into underlying causes may be provided by these difficult problems.

We have found a number of underlying causes occurring repeatedly, and the most common are listed here in their order of occurrence, starting with the most common.

Dysbiosis

This means the presence of abnormal bacteria, or the absence of normal bacteria in the colon. These patients often present with abdominal symptoms such as flatulence and disordered bowel habit. The causes of dysbiosis itself are many, but the most common are antibiotic therapy, debilitating illness of any kind and the consumption of refined diets. Normal bowel bacteria have a number of important functions, including the manufacture of vitamins. They are also important in maintaining the absorptive capacity of the lining of the bowel (the mucosa) at a normal level. If the bacteria are abnormal in any way the bowel mucosa becomes particularly absorptive, rather like a sieve in which the holes are too big. As a result toxins are reabsorbed from the bowel back into the circulation and foods enter the body in a partially digested state. The treatment of dysbiosis rests on normalizing the bowel bacteria, using live preparations of specific bacteria, and giving herbal or homoeopathic mixtures directed at restoring the liver and pancreas to normal function (these organs appear to be nearly always functioning at less than normal levels in patients with food sensitivities and dysbiosis).

Chemical toxicity

An increasing number of patients become sensitive following toxic exposure to chemicals. The most common culprits are insecticides, herbicides and weedkillers used in commercial crop spraying. Some patients are very sensitive to food additives as well as pesticide residues on food. Toxic chemicals tend to be deposited in fat cells, and therefore blood and urine tests are normal in these cases of slow insidious poisoning. This important fact has not been recognized, with the result that millions are being chronically poisoned; successful treatment is not easy in these cases. In our experience the best results have followed a sophisticated homoeopathic approach using homoeopathic dilutions of the toxins (known as nosodes) together with carefully chosen accompanying remedies. Regular exercise also helps the body to expel toxins.

Viral infections
Many patients give a history of never recovering from influenza or other viral infection. Often the initial illness is vague and undefined; however, sometimes it is more specific, with a definite diagnosis such as glandular fever having been made. A sophisticated application of homoeopathy as described under chemical toxicity is, in our view, the most successful approach in such cases.

Vitamin and mineral deficiency
Appropriate vitamin and mineral replacement as determined by hair analysis (see Chapter 10) can give marked improvement in some cases of multiple food and chemical sensitivity. In our view blind multiple vitamin and mineral therapy is inexcusable in severe cases of multiple sensitivity when excellent techniques such as hair analysis are available for monitoring body mineral levels. There is some evidence that much vitamin and mineral deficiency is due to the consumption of processed ('junk') foods.

Radiation from various sources
A small proportion of patients with multiple sensitivities are ill due to living or working in unsafe electrical environments. This can range from living near to high-voltage power lines to working with electrical equipment. The mechanism of action of these factors is unclear but seems to be related to the excess positive ionization produced by these installations. The treatment is either to move house or change jobs.

Psychological causes
Ecology has been the salvation of many patients whose illness has been labelled as being 'all in the mind', but this is a two-edged sword as it attracts patients whose problems are genuinely psychological. Unfortunately, these patients are doubly difficult to convince of the primary cause of their problems. In our experience the most successful treatment has been along psychotherapeutic lines.

Adulterated food, a cause of food sensitivity?

A dominant theme of the 'back to nature' movement is that chemical contamination of food is harmful and can cause multiple sensitivities, amongst other things. Contamination occurs in two main areas: the first is herbicide, pesticide and weedkiller residues on fruit and vegetables and the presence of traces of synthetic hormones and antibiotics in meat. The second is the addition of chemicals to foods in order to improve their shelf life, their texture (emulsifiers, etc.), or their appearance and therefore saleability (colourants, etc.).

There is some clinical evidence, albeit anecdotal at the time of writing, that the first group (herbicides, etc.) of food contamination can sometimes produce multiple sensitivities if the exposure is big enough. In practice this rarely happens, dangerous exposure to chemicals usually occurring during crop spraying or living near to areas of intensive agriculture. There is very little evidence that the second group of contamination of food with chemicals causes multiple sensitivities. There are, however, an increasing number of people who react to many chemicals in foods from both of the groups mentioned. In the vast majority of cases these are contributory rather than causative in the patient's problem.

On the other side of the coin the evidence that food processing seriously affects the nutritional value of food is overwhelming. A glance at the 'nutritional standards and composition of foods' section of the *Geigy Scientific Tables*, Volume 1 (8th Edition published by Ciba-Geigy Ltd, Basle, Switzerland), reveals that food processing has two major effects. First, it usually changes and often reverses the sodium/potassium ratio in foods. In the natural state most fruits and vegetables contain high levels of potassium and low levels of sodium. The body is very good indeed at conserving sodium and therefore requires very little (a high salt intake is a major health hazard and is all too common in the civilized world); in contrast it is bad at conserving potassium and loses this vital element with alarming ease. Therefore a high potassium and low sodium diet is a necessity. To give an example of the foregoing, the sodium/potassium ratio of fresh tomatoes is 3/268; for tinned tomatoes this changes to 130/217. The sodium/potassium ratio of cornflour is 1/120, but when corn is made into cornflakes the same ratio changes to 1160/120.

The second major effect of food processing is a major reduction in the vitamin content of the food, in some cases by a factor of ten times and in most cases by at least a half. It is therefore possible to become vitamin deficient in the midst of plenty. In our experience this is not uncommon and this subject is dealt with more extensively in the chapter on hair analysis. The wise will grow as much of their own food as possible, as this is the only way of guaranteeing freedom from contamination.

What is the mechanism of food and chemical sensitivity?
This topic is a minefield of controversy, ranging from the hard-line allergist who if there isn't a demonstrable immunological reaction going on considers that it doesn't exist, to the science-fiction approach which considers that some sort of ill-understood radiation is coming from the food or chemical and it is this to which the patient is reacting. There are many shades of opinion between these two extremes. It is useful to discuss some of the more unusual theories as conventional immunology falls seriously short of explaining the majority of food and chemical sensitivity reactions. Immunological reactions to food and chemicals have been described elsewhere in this book. Two possible modes of action will be discussed here; one is pharmacological and the other we have described as a radiation theory.

Pharmacological reactions
These reactions are due to the observation that many foods contain biologically active chemicals, particularly of the amine group. A good example is the presence of large amounts of tyramine (a commonly occurring amine) in chocolate and cheese. These foods can produce symptoms in susceptible individuals, often a migraine, by a pharmacological action rather like that of a drug.

Radiation theory
A number of clinical observations have led us to surmise that another as yet undiscovered but important mechanism is at work in food and chemical sensitivity. For example, when testing sensitive patients with the auriculo-cardiac reflex or Vega testing (see Chapter 8), a number develop symptoms during testing simply by having the substance placed near to them (when using the ACR), or in circuit with them (when using the Vegatest method), without in either case the substance having been in direct physical contact with

the patient. This phenomenon has been noted repeatedly by us and by many doctors to whom we have taught these testing methods. We are convinced that it is real and worthy of further investigation. One of us (JNK) is currently researching ways of photographing electromagnetic events around the body in order to try and develop a coherent and scientific account of these phenomena.

An interesting experience related to us by a medical colleague working in ecology is of relevance to the radiation hypothesis. It concerned a highly sensitive patient who, amongst other things, was sensitive to nickel. She claimed, to the utter disbelief of our colleague, that if any nickel-containing object was placed within a few feet of her then she would become ill as a result of reacting to it. My colleague, having an open-minded scientific approach, decided to test the patient in a blind fashion. The patient was blindfolded and she was led around the consulting rooms and asked to identify all nickel-containing objects simply by her physical proximity to them (not by direct physical contact). The patient got it right 100 per cent of the time.

We have observed a number of sensitive patients who claim that once they have eaten a sensitive food this contaminates all subsequent hitherto safe foods, often for the next few hours, and in some cases for the following three or four days. It is as if the unsafe food has radiated and contaminated all subsequent foods in the same way that a radioactive object will contaminate all surrounding, initially non-radioactive, objects.

It is easy to dismiss all of these phenomena as moonshine, and all too often they have been. They are worthy of investigation but demand much open-mindedness and courage on the part of the researcher trying to explain these observations. It is the unwillingness to look at the unexplained and to try novel solutions that is holding back furtherance of a real understanding of the important question of mechanisms of food and chemical sensitivity.

Conclusion

This chapter will have been of little interest to the average ecology patient who has got better by simple food avoidance. It will be of interest to the increasing number of patients who have relapsed following initial improvement from an ecological approach, or who are on a seemingly never-ending ecology merry-go-round of collecting more sensitivities and more switch-off drops. The ideas in this chapter at least offer these patients some hope of a fundamental cure, and therefore we have included it at the considered risk of confusing some readers, but stimulating others and hopefully helping yet more.

8. The Diagnosis and Management of Ecological Illness

DIAGNOSIS

The first question to answer in any illness which is thought to be wholly or partially ecological is whether symptoms disappear or at least improve on avoiding the offending foods and/or chemicals. If the patient's problem is due to foods, then fasting for at least five days should improve the symptoms and in some cases remove them altogether. If the illness is wholly or partially due to chemicals then different procedures will have to be followed, as will be discussed later. The principle of ecological diagnosis is to determine which foods and/or chemicals are responsible for the illness. There are a number of techniques in regular use in order to determine these.

Elimination dieting

This is the longest standing and probably most commonly used method of ecological diagnosis. The patient is asked to fast and drink spring water only for five days. Some practitioners allow the patient to eat foods which are rarely implicated in ecological illness, such as lamb, pears or kiwi fruit, etc. In our opinion a five-day, spring-water fast is the most effective method. It is interesting to note that similar fasting rituals form integral parts of some ancient systems of medicine such as Ayurvedic medicine. The implication of fasting in these systems of medicine is that it cleanses the body of toxins.

If symptoms are improved or disappear towards the end of the five-day fast, then it can be assumed that the patient's illness is due to one or a number of foods which he was eating. Symptoms often worsen on days two, three or four of the fast, a phenomenon reminiscent of a withdrawal reaction so commonly found when people try to stop smoking or when an alcoholic stops drinking. The majority of books about ecology stick to the five-day elimination diet as being the method of choice. In our view it has a number of limitations, the main one being that not all the symptoms will clear up after a five-day fast and a much longer period of avoidance may be necessary, particularly in rheumatoid arthritis. If a patient's symptoms are wholly or partially due to chemical exposure, then food elimination will often reveal nothing of any clinical use.

Following the five-day fast, the patient is told to reintroduce the foods he or she was previously eating, one at a time. The less commonly eaten foods should be reintroduced first and each meal should consist of only one food, such as eggs, fish, oranges, wheat, etc. If symptoms recur after a meal then the food taken is clearly implicated. This procedure is continued until all the foods have been introduced one by one, so that a list of food sensitivities is built up; it is important to remember that tap water should be considered as a food. It is usually adequate to reintroduce each food meal by meal rather than on a daily basis, as following the five-day fast the patient will be in the hypersensitive stage and therefore more likely to produce a rapid and definite reaction.

This method breaks down in those patients who react 24 hours following taking a food to which they are sensitive. The most delayed reaction we have encountered is one of 48 hours following taking an allergic food. Clearly, using an elimination dieting technique in these delayed reactors is a cumbersome and time-consuming procedure. The technique is cumbersome enough even in those who do react quickly on reintroduction of foods. The major drawback of this method, in our view, is that results are often confusing, and certainly not as clear (in some instances) as many ecology books lead one to believe. This is possibly due to a number of factors, not the least being that following such a rigorous regime requires an intelligent and highly motivated patient, as the disruption to lifestyle can be considerable when following an elimination diet. Also patients with ecological illness often have a collection of vague symptoms, such as depression or fatigue, and find it exceptionally difficult to decide whether they are fatigued or depressed following any particular food. In conclusion, we find that elimination dieting is a very useful technique, but with limited application due to the many practical problems which beset it.

The following techniques are methods of compiling a list of culprit foods and/or chemicals without the necessity for elimination dieting. In our experience a testing method of some sort is essential in order to manage ecological illness successfully, due to the apparent practical limitations of elimination dieting.

RAST

RAST stands for Radio Allergo Sorbent Test and is a method of locating specific antibodies in the blood serum to foods; in other words, it identifies true allergic reactions to foods. A recent leading article in the *British Medical Journal* (April, 1983) on food allergy cast doubt on the diagnostic value of RAST testing for food sensitivity; indeed, specific antibodies to common foods are often found in the serum of apparently non-food-allergic patients. There is little correlation between positive RAST followed by subsequent food avoidance of the implicated foods and clinical improvement of the patient. This interesting finding casts doubt on food sensitivity having an immunological basis. One other drawback of RAST, quite apart from its clinical irrelevance, is that the tests are expensive. Some doctors doggedly stick to RAST and are reluctant to admit of any sensitivity occurring outside of this testing procedure. This can be bad news for the frustrated patient who might find himself relegated to the psychological dustbin.

Cytotoxic testing

In this test, live white blood cells are exposed to a range of foods and chemicals. The presence or absence and degree of damage caused to these cells is an indicator of the presence of food and/or chemical sensitivity and gives some indication as to its degree. For example, if the white cells only increase in size and become rounded (they normally have an irregular shape) then this indicates a mild reaction. If the white cells burst this indicates a severe reaction. One of the many limitations of this test is that the presence and degree of white-cell damage is a matter of opinion on the part of the laboratory technician and often the results can be difficult to interpret. The correlation between food and/or chemical avoidance and clinical improvement is high for cytotoxic testing; this test is said to be approximately 80 per cent accurate. Its main disadvantages are that it often reveals too many sensitivities, usually more than thirty, and it is expensive. The average cost for testing fifty allergens is approximately £58 at the time of writing, but can go up to £135 for 144 different substances. It is, however, less expensive than RAST and is much more clinically useful.

Intradermal injection techniques

Intradermal injection testing means injecting tiny amounts (approximately four drops) of allergen just beneath the skin surface, raising a small round bump known as a wheal. A subsequent growth in the size of the wheal indicates a positive response and points to allergy. This is known as a positive whealing response; the technique is one of the diagnostic mainstays of conventional allergy. In practice these techniques are accurate indicators of allergy to airborne substances, such as pollens, dust, spores from moulds, etc., but are very poor at diagnosing allergy and/or sensitivity to foods or chemicals. Various authorities rate the diagnostic success of conventional intradermal testing for foods or chemicals as ranging from 18 to 40 per cent, hardly good enough to establish an accurate diagnosis. Perhaps the ones that are detected on conventional intradermal tests are true allergies, whilst those not detected in this way are sensitivities rather than allergies.

However, if the allergens are diluted with salt water in steps of five (i.e. dilution no. 1 is diluted 5 times, dilution no. 2 is diluted 25 times and so on) and these dilutions are injected intradermally, then reactions begin to appear. Often the patient develops symptoms related to their complaint, such as headache or abdominal pain, at the same time. For example, a patient may produce no positive whealing response to the injection of a wheat concentrate but if this is diluted in steps of five, then one of the dilutions — often the first — will produce a positive whealing response if the patient is sensitive to wheat. Within the framework of conventional allergy this phenomenon is inexplicable, i.e. no whealing on injection of a concentrate but a positive whealing response on injection of a dilution. Yet it is repeatedly observed and has been used by us in the past as a diagnostic technique with identical findings. A majority of patients (about 70 per cent) develop symptoms together with a positive whealing response. Increasing dilutions are usually injected at approximately half-hourly intervals until the dilution which produces no whealing (the so-called first negative wheal) is reached. This is often accompanied by an almost instantaneous 'switch-off' of symptoms. This dilution can then be used as a 'switch-off' drop to enable the patient to eat small amounts of the offending food after having first taken an appropriate 'switch-off' drop under the tongue. At the time of writing we have no explanation why a dilution of a substance can 'switch-off' a patient's reaction to that substance and this observation must join the host of unexplained observations made by clinical ecologists. The fact that the technique works at all remains something of an enigma to many ecologists. This technique has become known as the Miller technique after an American doctor, Dr Joe Miller, who first suggested it in the early 1960s.

The Miller technique therefore provides a diagnostic and therapeutic approach to ecology rolled into one, and is the mainstay of many ecology clinics, but unfortunately it has many disadvantages. It is very time-consuming and often encourages an unhealthy introspection on the part of the patient to his problem. Desensitization using this technique tends to be very specific (in other words it isn't possible to give one 'switch-off' drop for a group of related substances), so many substances need to be tested. Also some patients find that they continually develop new sensitivities. It is therefore a useful yet unwieldy diagnostic technique, and probably a less than perfect method for treating food and chemical sensitivity.

Clinical testing using the auricular cardiac reflex (ACR)

The ACR is a physical sign used in a branch of ear acupuncture known as auricular medicine, hence its odd-sounding name. First noticed by Dr Paul Nogier, it is a small movement of the position where the wrist pulse is strongest, either in the direction of the elbow (a so-called negative ACR) or in the direction of the wrist (a so-called positive ACR). It is not to be confused with the Coca pulse test which records an increase in pulse rate of ten or more beats following ingestion of an allergic-sensitive food. The ACR changes in response to small changes in the body's energy field. One of us (JNK) adapted this finding to ecology and noted that by bringing a dried food near to the body (within half an inch of the skin but not touching the skin), then the ACR changes.

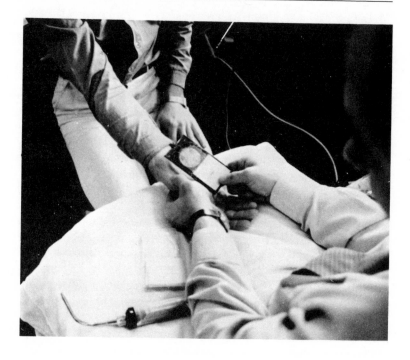

Figure 5:   Clinical testing using the ACR.

Depending on where on the body the food is brought up to then a diagnosis of which foods or chemicals the patient is sensitive to can be made (see Figure 5). It is hard to believe that bringing a substance near to the body, but without touching it, can cause a subtle change in that body. Some scientific backing comes for this technique from studying subtle electromagnetic change around the body using sensitive and highly sophisticated electronic monitoring equipment.

In experienced hands this test is approximately 80 per cent accurate (about the same as cytotoxic testing). Its advantages are that it is quick (fifty foods or chemicals can be tested in fifteen minutes), it only requires dried food samples mounted in specially prepared filters, and it is cheap. Its disadvantage is that it requires some training in order to be able to detect it accurately, and there are some doctors who find it impossible to learn — in the same way that some doctors find heart murmurs almost impossible to hear.

Electrical testing for food and chemical sensitivities (Vega testing)

The rapid 'switch-off' of symptoms, found when determining neutralizing drops using the Miller technique, has been observed by many doctors who have used this method. It has been surmised that the 'switch-off' is too rapid for it to have been mediated by a biochemical change in the body, and that an electrical mechanism of some sort is more likely. Not surprisingly, therefore, electrical testing for food and chemical sensitivities is a practical possibility. These methods owe their origin to electrical measurement techniques of acupuncture points and the observation that these measurements vary if a substance relevant to the patient is placed, inside a glass container, in series in the circuit (see Figure 6). This interesting phenomenon is difficult to explain using classical electromagnetic theory, yet it remains a useful method for testing either for therapy or diagnosis. It is used in ecology as a diagnostic method.

A normal reading is obtained over a specific acupuncture point, then a control substance in a glass bottle is introduced into the circuit — which should always lower the reading on subsequent

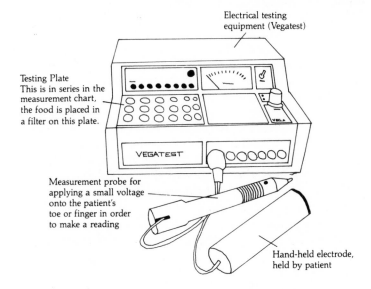

Figure 6: Electrical testing equipment (Vegatest).

measurement of the point. The control substance used is usually a poison of some sort, i.e. something that will harm the body if taken internally. Then each food or chemical is placed one by one on the testing plate and those that lower the reading are the ones to which the patient is sensitive. The method can also be used to determine desensitization end points. The advantages of this method are that it is quick, cheap to perform, and carries a certain placebo effect in that the patient can see the reading change on the meter when foods or chemicals to which he is sensitive are in circuit. Patients have confidence in this method, probably because of this effect, and they are therefore more likely to follow rigorous avoidance of the relevant foods or chemicals than when using other diagnostic methods.

Its disadvantages are that the equipment (a Vegatest device) required is expensive, although it represents a once-only purchase, and that the technique requires considerable skill in order to carry it out effectively. Like the ACR method, a small proportion of doctors are unable to use it effectively. In skilled hands it is approximately 80 per cent accurate.

Testing using Applied Kinesiology
This method assesses changes in muscle strength with hand contact of the suspected sensitive foods or chemicals. The food or chemical to be tested is placed in the hand of the subject to be tested and a muscle is chosen to assess any alteration in power due to the patient's contact with the test substance. A food or chemical to which the subject is sensitive will weaken muscle power, and those which the patient needs will strengthen it. The mechanism of action of this test is unclear but is likely to be similar to those of the ACR and electrical testing methods. Testing using Applied Kinesiology has been done on a double-blind basis (where neither the subject nor doctor knows the identity of the test substance) and has produced reliable and significant results.

Its advantages are that it is cheap and requires little equipment. One disadvantage in common with ACR and electrical testing is that it requires considerable skill on the part of the practitioner. It is also a more time-consuming method than ACR or electrical testing, but it shares the same level of accuracy as the ACR and electrical testing methods.

Conclusion

A number of testing methods are available of which the most reliable are, in skilled hands, cytotoxic testing, ACR, electrical testing and Applied Kinesiology. ACR, electrical testing and Applied Kinesiology win on grounds of cost and are therefore to be preferred. In our view the best method is the electrical testing because of the placebo effect of the testing instrument.

Food and chemical testing, particularly cytotoxic testing, has come in for considerable criticism on the grounds that the tests are not repeatable; in other words, slightly different results may be obtained on subsequent retesting. However, the key sensitivities always come up again on subsequent testing. In our view the reason for this is that sensitivities do in fact change within broad limits. The more severe a patient's problem then the quicker the sensitivities change, i.e. the patient is in a very labile state. Therefore complete duplication of these test results should not be expected.

TREATMENT

Once a clear diagnosis has been made in terms of which foods and chemicals to avoid, the battle is largely won. Treatment is either by food avoidance and rotation dieting or desensitization.

Food avoidance and rotation diets

The simplest approach is to exclude the sensitive foods from the diet. It is important to vary the remaining foods as much as possible, and the system for doing this is called rotation dieting. This means not eating one food within three days of having eaten it previously (a three-day rotation) or sometimes a seven-day rotation is recommended (i.e. not eating a food within seven days of having previously eaten it). The longer the rotation then the more difficult it is to design. The idea of rotation dieting is to minimize the chances of developing sensitivities to new foods. The majority of food sensitive patients manage very satisfactorily on simple avoidance and rotation dieting; however, in very sensitive patients this simple approach to treatment breaks down.

As a general rule, once the foods to which the patient has been sensitive have been avoided for six to nine months they can be carefully reintroduced into a rotation dieting plan. At this stage the average patient has developed tolerance to these foods, but if they are eaten with anything like the regularity they were before food avoidance, then masked sensitivity will develop again. Some food sensitivities appear to be fixed, in that tolerance never develops. This is perhaps due to lack of essential enzymes in particular patients to cope with these foods. The best example is lactase deficiency for digesting milk and dairy products; this is commonly seen in Negro and Oriental races.

Some practitioners recommend rotating food families as well as individual foods: for example, potatoes and tomatoes belong to the same family and therefore shouldn't be eaten within three days of each other on a three-day rotation.

Desensitization

This has been described in some detail in the section on intradermal injection techniques. The principle is to find a dilution of the food or chemical to which the patient is sensitive which will switch the reaction off to the relevant substance. Generally speaking, the 'switch off' is given in the form of drops which are dropped under the tongue approximately ten minutes before exposure to the food or chemical. Only one drop is required, and cocktails may be made containing many food and chemical 'switch off' drops all mixed together. Some practitioners recommend 'switch offs' by intradermal injection, claiming that these produce a long-lasting effect of two-three days, and that they are more effective than sublingual drops. Sublingual drops only work for a few hours and therefore have to be taken at least three times daily if exposure to the food or chemical is occurring regularly; in some instances drops may have to be taken hourly if exposure is particularly heavy, such as to gas or petrol fumes. In our experience intradermal injection of 'switch off' drops does produce longer lasting symptom relief than sublingual drops, but we have not found that intradermal injections are any more effective than by using the sublingual route. We therefore use the sublingual route exclusively as it is more convenient.

Methods of locating the 'switch off' end point

A number of methods can be used to find the dilution which switches the patient's reaction off. The most commonly used is the intradermal injection technique described by Dr Joe Miller. The ACR, electrical testing using the Vega apparatus or Applied Kinesiology can also be used. The major disadvantages of the intradermal technique are that it is time consuming (in our hands it takes approximately forty minutes to determine one end point) and that the symptoms it produces during a testing session can be difficult to reverse in very sensitive patients. The other three methods are quick and don't cause symptoms in the patient except in the most sensitive cases. In our view electrical testing is the best and most accurate method; an end point can be determined in approximately three minutes using this technique. The disadvantage is that considerable skill on the part of the practitioner is needed.

Mechanism of action of desensitization

The mode of action of ecological desensitization is unclear. In our opinion an electrical mechanism of an ill-understood nature is involved as the 'switch off' often occurs rapidly following a single sublingual drop. It surprises us that this method of desensitization seems to have been accepted uncritically by many doctors practising ecology, as it has many parallels with homoeopathy, a healing art which continues to attract derision from the majority of doctors, including some ecologists.

Uses of desensitization

Desensitization is useful for patients who cannot follow a strict diet due to pressures of a busy life or a difficult home environment. It is essential in patients who are so multiply sensitive that their safe diet is nutritionally inadequate. Desensitization at least allows these patients to expand their diets and thereby maintain adequate nutrition. Patients who are chemically sensitive, particularly to airborne chemicals, need desensitization if they are going to lead a reasonable existence in an urban environment. It is impossible to avoid petrol or diesel fumes in this situation. Therefore desensitization offers some hope for these patients who, for reasons of job or family commitments, are unable to make sufficiently rigorous environmental changes to avoid exposure to airborne chemicals.

Return of symptoms whilst taking desensitization drops

Some patients develop symptoms again after having been successfully 'switched off' to the foods and chemicals to which they were sensitive. This is usually due to a change in the 'switch off' point, but can be due to the development of another sensitivity.

This means that patients on 'switch off' drops need their end points checking periodically. If intradermal injection is used to determine 'switch offs', then this can be an expensive procedure. As yet none of these methods is widely available within the NHS yet; clearly, cheaper techniques such as the ACR or electrical testing are more suitable in a health-service situation.

For how long does desensitization need to be continued?

The average patient with ecological illness loses his sensitivities following a prolonged period of avoidance, usually in the order of two to three years. Sublingual desensitization usually shortens this time to two years — or even eighteen months in some cases — when often the patient can gradually come off drops and tolerate moderate intermittent exposure to the previously sensitive foods and chemicals.

Disadvantages of desensitization

Desensitization is by no means always successful. The more sensitive a patient, the less likely it is that it offers a practical solution. Often in these patients, end points change rapidly, in some cases almost daily, and it becomes impractical to keep changing end points. Some patients on desensitization have an alarming tendency to develop more sensitivities, and in our experience desensitization may accelerate this tendency amongst the most sensitive patients.

Enzyme potentiated desensitization (EPD)

This is a method for treating allergies which has been developed by Dr Len McEwan, originally of St Mary's Hospital Medical School, London and latterly from the London Medical Centre. The method consists of placing a mixture of highly purified antigens, in very small doses indeed, with an enzyme called β-glucuronidase to potentiate the effect of the antigens mixed together with two other chemicals.

A small plastic cup containing the appropriate desensitizing fluid is placed over an area of skin which has previously been scarified using a blunt scalpel (see Figure 7). This cup is left in place for 24 hours; however, if a severe reaction develops, which in our experience does happen with some regularity in very sensitive patients, then the patient can remove the cup earlier.

It is possible to apply a standard mixture of more than seventy

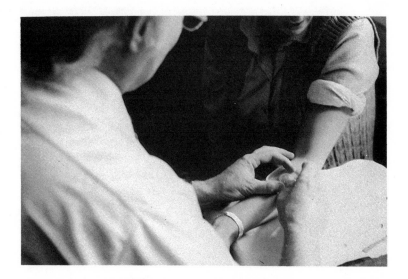

Figure 7: A small plastic cup is placed over the forearm skin.

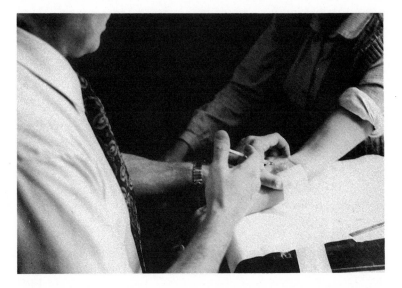

Figure 7a: The antigen mixture (usually a mixture of a number of foods, sometimes pollens or molds are added) is injected into the plastic cup.

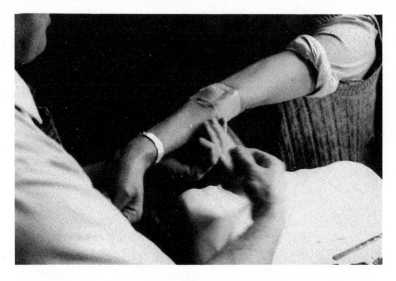

Figure 7b: The plastic cup is then fixed to the arm using tape and is left there for twenty-four hours after which time it is removed.

allergens, in the hope that all the important ones have been included. So it is not essential to identify all the patient's sensitivities. The tendency to develop new sensitivities seen so often in sublingual drop desensitization is not apparent with this method. These factors give it obvious advantages over the 'switch off' drop method.

Treatment is usually given monthly for three months, with booster doses every four months. The average patient with multiple food sensitivities can expect to develop tolerance to his sensitive foods in six to twelve months from starting treatment — unlike desensitization drops, it doesn't work immediately. To date, this method is not widely available and so far as we know is not offered within the Health Service. Like sublingual drop desensitization it is much less useful in the patient with multiple sensitivities.

Conclusion
The simplest method of ecological treatment is avoidance. Many patients respond well to this approach. Desensitization enables patients with multiple sensitivities to live a more normal life. EPD takes longer to produce a result, but probably produces a better result in a shorter time for the average patient. The limitations of each approach have been discussed.

9. Chemical Sensitivity

Chemical sensitivity is becoming an increasingly important aspect of ecology. The existence of chemical sensitivity was first noted by an American doctor, Dr Albert Rowe, in the 1930s. He noticed that some of his patients reacted to apples which had been sprayed with pesticides but not to ones taken from unsprayed orchards. He noticed that this phenomenon spread to other fruits, and in true transatlantic style he gave it a name — 'multiple fruit sensitivity'. This started a growing awareness that pesticides, weedkillers and herbicides aren't the only ecologically harmful chemicals, but also many seemingly innocuous hydrocarbon products which all of us have strewn around our homes, are deadly poisons to some. Current thinking in ecology is that chemical and hydrocarbon sensitivity is as important and environmentally far more worrying than food sensitivity. This area of ecology is much more difficult to diagnose clinically with anything like the accuracy of specific food sensitivities, as often the patient has little choice or knowledge as to whether he or she is exposed or not to a multitude of airborne chemicals. A testing method of some sort is essential to be able to manage chemical sensitivities effectively.

Generally speaking, chemical sensitivity goes hand in hand with food sensitivity. In some patients the chemical and hydrocarbon sensitivity predominates over the food sensitivity, in others foods are more important. It is usually possible to sort out the majority of ecological problems concentrating on foods alone, but unfortunately this situation is changing, particularly for the most sensitive people, and for these it is necessary to unravel the tangle of hydrocarbon and chemical exposure in order to achieve a reasonable clinical result.

The outlook for the future is bleak, as there are no signs that hydrocarbon, pesticide, food additive, and aerosol propellant pollution is on the decrease; if anything, it is increasing. The most important chemical sensitivity is to hydrocarbons, particularly petrol, diesel and gas.

Hydrocarbon sensitivity

People with hydrocarbon sensitivity often complain of what the Americans call 'brain fag'. This describes an intermittent state of varying severity (depending on the level of exposure) of mental confusion, poor memory, slurring of speech and a general dulling of all the senses, particularly sight. These symptoms can be caused by other sensitivities but they are most commonly associated with hydrocarbon sensitivity.

The clue as to whether the patient is sensitive to these substances comes from the history: for example, the patient who goes to sleep sitting in front of a gas fire or near to a mobile calor gas heater, but isn't so affected when sitting in front of an electric fire; the patient who suffers from car sickness, the motorist who constantly has to fight extreme fatigue when motorway driving. All these suggest hydrocarbon sensitivity. Usually these people have an acute sense of smell to minute amounts of gas or petrol fumes, but some of the most severely affected cases eventually lose all sense of smell.

How does the patient sort out these problems? Exposure can certainly be minimized. Getting rid of gas stoves and gas fires is a good first step, while for petrol-sensitive patients travelling in the front of the car where fumes are less can be helpful. A filter fitted to the car heater is also worth considering, as an unfiltered heater simply blows other vehicles' exhaust fumes into the car. Some Japanese cars have these fitted as standard.

Patients who react strongly to gas may need to go to the lengths of having all gas pipes as well as gas boilers, cookers and fires removed from the house. Even cooking pans and utensils that have been used over a gas stove may also need to be removed. This might sound like taking things too far, but any doctor who has been confronted by severely gas-sensitive patients would be the first to concur with the usefulness of such apparently draconian advice.

Desensitization is clearly useful in these patients, as it means that they are able to cope with a level of exposure which is beyond their control. Many people cannot afford the measures suggested to create an ecologically safe haven for themselves. Desensitization can be a more manageable alternative for these people, although we have some doubts as to whether this is the best approach in the long term. Hydrocarbon-sensitive people are advised to use electric heating instead of oil- or gas-fired central heating, even though the boiler may be situated outside the house.

Hydrocarbon derivatives
Substances derived from hydrocarbons are legion, and often patients who are sensitive to gas, petrol and diesel are also sensitive to many hydrocarbon derivatives.

Plastics
Articles made from hydrocarbon derivatives, particularly plastics, can affect hydrocarbon-sensitive patients. Soft plastics of all types should be avoided. Storing food in Tupperware-type containers will contaminate the food for these sensitive patients — glass storage jars are the safest method of food storage. Hard plastics such as Bakelite are usually safe and don't give off fumes in the same way that polythene does. Some people react to plastic glasses with sore, running eyes and irritation of the eyelids. These people should obtain steel rimmed glasses with the lenses free of plastic coating (many spectacle lenses are covered with a protective plastic film).

Synthetic clothing
Severely hydrocarbon-sensitive patients should also take steps to avoid all close contact with hydrocarbon derivatives, particularly clothing. This therefore means dressing in clothes made from natural materials such as wool or cotton; and in practice these can be very difficult to obtain, as a mixture of 70 per cent wool or cotton with the rest being a man-made fibre is generally the purest that can be obtained. For such patients it is very well worth searching to obtain pure wool or pure cotton garments, since nylon and many other man-made fibres are derived wholly or in part from hydrocarbons. This sort of attention to detail will produce enormous dividends to the health of these patients.

Other hydrocarbon derivatives
This covers a large group of substances, but the following list contains the main ones:

Paints   Wax candles
Varnishes   Coal fires
Solvents   Air fresheners
Cleaning fluids   Deodorants
Lighter fuel   Disinfectants, especially
Propellants in aerosol sprays   pine-scented ones
Coal-tar soaps   Cosmetics
Detergents   Perfumes
Polishes   Sponge rubber

Multiply chemically sensitive patients should be advised on avoidance of all the items in the above list. Hypo-allergenic all-purpose cleaning materials are now made by an American company called Shaklee, whose products are becoming more widely available in Britain through health-food shops. They may be obtained through most health food shops. Women are often resistant to the idea of stopping using cosmetics and perfumes, but if successfully persuaded the results in terms of improved health are often gratifying.

Phenol
Phenol, rather like hydrocarbons, is a ubiquitous chemical. It is contained in the following substances:

Carbolic is phenol   Preservatives in allergy
Herbicides   antigen solutions
Pesticides   In manufacture of:
Bakelite   epoxy and phenoxic resins
Moulded articles, like   aspirin and other drugs
    telephones   nylon
Synthetic detergents   polyurethane
Petrol (traffic fumes)   explosives
Dyes   Casing of electric wiring
Photographic solutions   and cables
Preservatives in   Perfumes
    medications

Formalin

Formalin is similar to phenol in that it is widespread and people are often sensitive to it. It is contained in the following substances:

Traffic fumes
Glues and cements
Matches
Foam rubber — a synthetic,
  used in:
  furniture and pillows
  mattresses
  foam-backed curtains and
    carpets
All propellants (sprays)
Softlan and other fabric
  softeners/conditioners
Hospitals:
  orthopaedic casts
  hospital sick rooms
  surgical instrument
    cleaning
Manufacture of vitamins A
  and E
All textiles:
  dyes
  permanent-press treatment
  wrinkle-resisting
    treatment
  mildew proofing
  water-repellant treatment
  shrink-proofing
  moth-proofing
  stretch fabrics
Paper manufacture
Newspaper and newsprint
Photography and
  photographs
Butter and cheese
All UK dairy milk

Milk products:
  powdered cream, milk
    puddings, etc.
Antiperspirants
Disinfectants
Dentifrice antiseptics
Mouthwashes
Nail polishes
Toothpastes
Insecticides
Fertilizers
Tanning agent in tanning
  of animal skins
Soft plastics
Soaps — germicidal
  detergents
  shampoos
Hair-setting lotion
Air deodorants
Waste incineration
Building materials:
  concrete
  plaster
  wallboard
  synthetic resins
  wood veneers
  wood preservatives
Cavity-wall insulation
Used in the manufacture of
  antibiotics
Polluted air:
  smog
  petrol and diesel fumes
    which cause burning
    eyes, etc.

Chemical pollution of meat

Practically all meat available in the average butcher's shop has been intensively reared and generally contains trace levels of antibiotics and in some cases other drugs, which have been given to the animals. Some very sensitive patients react to meat, and indeed to many foods, simply because of the contaminants that these foods contain. Our experience has convinced us that if these patients can obtain and eat organic (uncontaminated) food then they can often tolerate these foods with no reaction at all. Uncontaminated meat is only available from a small number of farmers who specialize in producing it, or by eating wild game. All of these food sources are relatively expensive. Patients who are financially stretched should be advised to become vegetarian and grow as much of their own food as possible. Unfortunately this is not entirely free from danger, as a recent study on lead levels in vegetables has shown, the findings being that vegetables, particularly brassicas, grown within a ten-mile radius of central London, contain unacceptably high levels of lead due to atmospheric pollution. Perhaps the abolition of lead in petrol may help to reverse this sad situation.

Food colourants

The addition of colourants to processed foods is common practice as this makes the food look attractive and therefore more easily saleable. Frozen peas often look almost luminous; orange squash looks bright orange. Whilst looking attractive to the eye they can play havoc with some patients: disorders of the nervous system, particularly hyperactivity in children, have been closely associated with reaction to colourants, in particular tartrazine (an orange colourant). Tartrazine has also been associated with childhood asthma. These connections have been recognized in the United States where tartrazine is banned, but ironically many children's medicines contain added colourant, often making the sensitive child worse. Parents of such children are well advised to ask for colourless medicine.

Colourants probably have a pharmacological (drug-like) effect on sensitive individuals as they seem to have a predilection for nerve synapses (these are the relay stations in the nervous system where one nerve ends and another begins). Highly complex neurochemical reactions occur at synapses (this is a small gap or cleft between the end of one nerve and the beginning of the next across which a number of chemical substances pass) and these processes are highly sensitive to modulation by any chemical which happens to be around. Colourants seem to be just such a group of compounds which can modulate synaptic transmission of nerve impulses, often facilitating this transmission and therefore producing hyperactivity. The only effective treatment for colourant sensitivity is avoidance.

The following list shows foods to which artificial colourants are commonly added:

Crème de menthe
Glacé cherries or other coloured fruits
Coloured ice-creams
Coloured sweets
Some cheeses
Butter
Margarine
Artificial orange squashes
Coca-cola and other coloured soft drinks
Many processed foods

Drugs
Sensitivity to drugs is more widespread than the medical profession likes to think. Recent evidence has found a possible connection between patients who react to many drugs and an enzyme deficiency. This means that some people, because of an enzyme deficiency, deal with drugs in a different way to normal people; but in spite of this finding it doesn't tell us how to prevent this happening. It is therefore wise for patients with multiple sensitivities to take as few drugs as possible, and to try and obtain treatment using an alternative therapy which has fewer side-effects than drug therapy. It is important to maintain a balanced view when discussing modern drug therapy, as its 'popular face' leads one to suspect that all drug therapy is bad. This is far from the truth, as many modern drugs are life-savers — antibiotics and anticoagulants being two obvious examples. Many others are obviously harmful and potentially lethal. As long as patients receive medical advice which reflects an unprejudiced view of both alternative and modern drug approaches then they have little to fear.

Tap-water sensitivity

Tap water contains a vast array of chemicals, the most dangerous being lead, cadmium and nitrates (derived from fertilizers used in agriculture). Norms of upper limits of these chemicals are clearly defined for many constituents of tap water, yet in our experience an alarming number of patients with ecological illness react to it. This raises the question as to what upper limits of normal mean; for whom do they apply? They certainly don't apply to the sensitive patient.

Most people who react to tap water do so following drinking it; a few also react when they wash in it, particularly patients with eczema. The treatment is to avoid tap water and drink bottled spring water, or to collect rain water from the roof of the house using a galvanized iron container (such as a bin or an old loft-type water collection tank); plastic tanks of any sort will not do. Rain-water collection in central city areas or near to large industrial complexes such as oil refineries or chemical-processing plants is likely to be less than pure. These people will have to rely on bottled spring water. Otherwise rain water is to be preferred on grounds of cost and ready availability. We have both noted remarkable improvements in patients following a change to rain water.

Filtering tap water is another possibility but isn't anything like as effective as using rain water. A simple, cheap, water filter is made by the Brita company and is available at a number of large chemists and health-food shops. More sophisticated water filters are available from Culligan International Company, High Wycombe, Buckinghamshire, UK.

Sensitivity to soap and detergents

This is often a forgotten part of the ecological history. An obvious piece of advice is that all so-called biological washing powders should be avoided. Ecologically safe washing powders are made by the Shaklee company.

All coal-tar derived soaps should be looked upon with suspicion, as must any scented soap, particularly pine-scented.

Smoking

Nearly all chemically sensitive patients are sensitive to cigarettes, cigar and pipe smoke. If they smoke they should make every effort to stop. They should also avoid crowded, smoke-filled places such as pubs, some restaurants and smoking compartments in trains.

What can be done for the Multiply Chemically Sensitive Patient?

1 *Avoidance*
The best approach is avoidance and the creation of an ecologically safe haven, both at home and at work. If the advice given in this chapter is followed then the reactions to chemicals can be reduced to a minimum.

A useful additional idea is the use of a portable air filter (a number of companies make sufficiently powerful filters, such as Patent Filtration Limited, Richmond, Surrey, UK) for people reacting to airborne chemicals. Often the use of a filter alone can produce a dramatic improvement in some patients.

Smokers who have multiple sensitivities must stop smoking, as must the people with whom they live.

2 *Desensitization*
Desensitization procedures are an important means of helping people with chemical sensitivity. The most common chemicals we switch off for are: gas, petrol, diesel, paint fumes (terpenes), ethanol, phenol, formalin, butane, propane and calor gas. Some ecologists claim that desensitization with ethanol and phenol dilutions will switch reactions off to the whole range of hydrocarbons. In our experience this is rarely the case, and it is usually necessary to desensitize to specific chemicals as indicated above. This is a disadvantage of desensitization, in that it tends to be very specific for particular chemicals.

Unfortunately, many patients with severe chemical sensitivity do not desensitize well, as their end points change with alarming rapidity. It is important to look for underlying causes in these people.

3 *The ecology unit*
American clinical ecologists have built a number of allergy-free in-patient units, where every possible detail has been thought of, right down to the paint on the walls and the air in the rooms. Nobody wearing perfume or aftershave is allowed in. Severely sensitive patients are admitted to these units in an attempt to remove all possible allergic contact. The aim is to see whether the patient

improves, as the sort of chemical avoidance possible in an ecology unit is far beyond anything that the patient can contrive in his own home.

Even though ecology units sound and look like modern technological wonders, they have a number of important drawbacks. The first is that they are exorbitantly expensive to stay in because of the minute attention to possible chemical exposure which is needed. Second, it is debatable as to how useful it is to demonstrate that a patient is multiply food and chemically sensitive without answering the question of what to do about it. Lastly, severely sensitive patients are badly maladapted to their environment, a situation solved in an ecology unit by radically changing the environment, but which cannot go on for ever and tends to maintain the patient in a maladapted state. Our view is that it is more useful and sensible to concentrate on measures such as a search for underlying causes and treating them, or vitamin and mineral replacement so as to help the patient adapt better to an imperfect environment.

Total allergy

Ecologists have been taunted by their orthodox colleagues by the presumed existence (by ecologists) of patients with total allergy. Doctors, generally with no experience of ecology, refuse to countenance that anybody could become sensitive to the majority of foods and chemicals, a surprisingly unscientific stance. Many patients are also unable to accept this idea for similar reasons. The truth in our view is somewhat different, as there are a small number of patients who react to the majority of foods and chemicals, giving a clinical picture of total allergy — to pretend that this doesn't exist doesn't help the patient. To think the problem is due to overbreathing, as suggested by a well-known British doctor, is less than useful. (The treatment for this is for the patient to breathe from a paper bag over the face to increase blood levels of carbon dioxide; this uniformly has no effect on these patients.) In a number of instances 'total allergy' is used as an excuse for severe personality disorders. This does not decry the existence of total allergy, but it does require considerable clinical skill to resolve this problem successfully.

The treatment of total allergy is long and laborious and should concentrate on making an ecologically safe haven with organically grown foods readily available and/or to define and treat the underlying causes. Desensitization is uniformly disappointing in these cases. Total allergy is getting more common, so a recognition of its existence is of some importance for us to be able to find out anything more about this life-threatening condition.

10. Hair Analysis and Trace Mineral Analysis

If a large animal becomes ill, then one investigation frequently used by vets is to burn a tiny sample of its hair and analyse it spectrophotometrically for trace metal content. Treatment often involves the use of specialized salt licks or other forms of mineral replacement. Hair is a body tissue, and one that is simple and painless to obtain for analysis. Most medical investigations in humans are based on blood analyses; the concentration of most chemicals, and in particular minerals, in the blood is dependent on many variables and the balancing mechanisms of the body tend to maintain blood levels at the cost of depleting the tissues of minerals. There is good evidence to suggest that a tissue estimation is, on the whole, a safer more stable and more accurate method of evaluating total body mineral content. The test is objective, easy to repeat, cheap and available and yet it is an investigation almost unheard of within conventional medicine.

The reason for the conspicuous absence of hair analysis in day-to-day medicine is probably based on ignorance of its existence and a lack of the simple information required to interpret the data correctly. Nevertheless the test is a useful one, particularly within the context of a practice that involves clinical ecology.

One of the major reasons for using this information within an ecological practice is that gross abnormalities in trace metals (mineral poisoning or deficiency) may well represent the trigger for multiple sensitivity. If the body is knocked 'off centre', it is far less able to cope with the stresses and toxins in the form of food and/or chemicals. Knowing whether there is a tissue lack or excess of particular minerals enables an accurate diagnosis to be made and any abnormalities to be corrected.

Trace metals are an essential factor in our normal metabolism; for instance zinc is vital for normal fertility and wound healing and also for the manufacture and metabolism of insulin by the pancreas. Iron is an essential oxygen-carrying molecule in blood, calcium is one of the most important metals that goes to make up healthy bones, and sodium and potassium are vital in the simple energetic processes that go on in all healthy living tissue. Gross disturbances of the tissue levels of these metals *must* result in serious bodily malfunction. Some of the common problems involve copper, zinc, lead and chromium.

Copper

An excess of copper in the tissues occurs quite frequently, particularly in young women who have been taking oral contraceptives or who have a copper intra-uterine contraceptive device. The female hormones in the oral contraceptive pill displace copper from the blood and deposit it in the tissues (such as hair), leading to a cellular overload of copper. This quite definitely predisposes a susceptible group of the population to the development of multiple and severe sensitivities that will frequently remain unresolved until the copper level is brought back to normal.

The simplest way to decrease high copper is to stop further contact with copper. Such measures would include:

1   Check the copper content of tap water and filter it if it is high in copper (use a public analyst to check this). Substitution with rain water is the safest solution in the worst cases.
2   Stop the oral contraceptive or remove any copper intra-uterine contraceptive device.
3   Check cooking implements such as copper pans; either make sure the copper pans are properly tinned or don't use them.

These measures should stop further absorption of copper. The copper can then be removed from the tissues over a period of about six months by chelating the high copper out with homoeopathic doses of copper. We recommend the use of Cuprum Metallicum in 200c strength, one tablet twice a week for six months and then

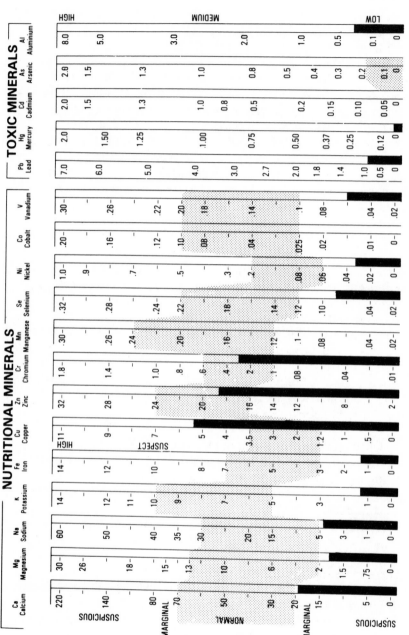

Figure 8: Hair analysis showing high copper level.

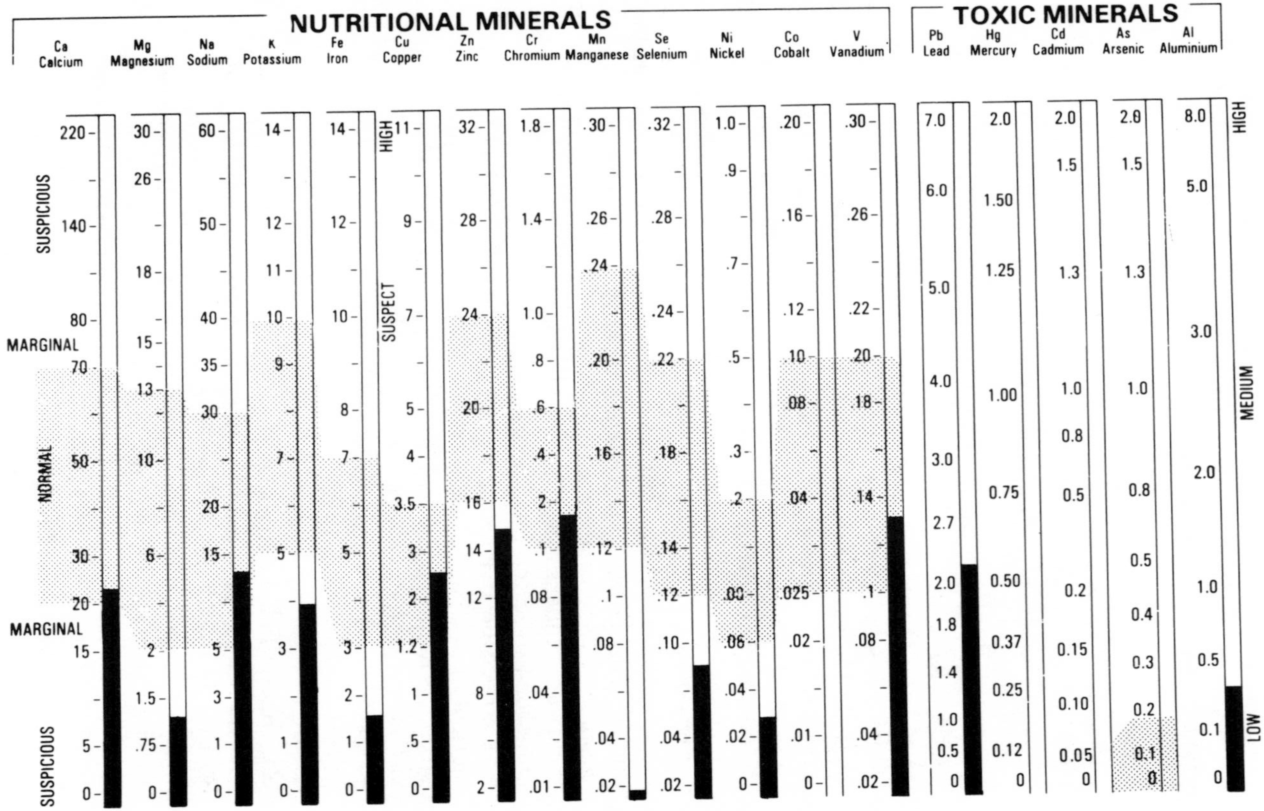

NUTRITIONAL MINERALS / TOXIC MINERALS

Figure 9: Hair analysis showing high lead level.

re-analyse the hair about nine months after the first analysis; during this period of time the copper content should drop with the homoeopathic medication alone.

Lead

There has been considerable public debate about the emission of lead from car exhausts. Most of the evidence available is hinged around blood lead levels; good arguments have been put forward which suggest that hair lead levels provide a better estimate of the tissue content of lead. In our opinion mild lead poisoning is endemic in the UK.

High lead levels seem to underlie many situations where multiple sensitivities are a problem. The hair analysis shown in Figure 9 is that of a young girl with severe eczema, which had not been responding to food exclusion. However, when the lead levels were controlled over about six months with homoeopathic doses of lead (Plumbum Metallicum 200c, one tablet twice a week) she began to respond to a food-exclusion diet, her hair lead level began to come down and she felt much better in herself. The cause of the high lead levels seem to have been directly attributable to the lead piping in her house, which is a grand old Victorian structure, but has not had any significant changes in its plumbing since it was built. Consequently if a high lead level is identified then it is important to search for potential sources of contamination.

It is probable that her blood levels would have been within the normal range. The *last* thing to become abnormal in almost any stressed situation is the blood level of minerals. Tissue excess or deficiency is the first indicator of problems and may result in symptoms, even though blood levels remain normal.

Zinc

Zinc has for many years been a fashionable method of promoting wound healing, and many local applications for external ulcers involve the use of zinc ointments or pastes. Although this therapy is now no longer widely used, there is some good evidence to suggest that low body zinc levels may well be of considerable importance. Studies of zinc levels in rats have clearly demonstrated that even mildly low tissue zinc levels result in difficult deliveries and severe behavioural abnormalities, both in the mother and baby rat. Rat diets severely deficient in zinc results in lethargy, malaise and severely impaired learning performance. To a certain extent this information has been confirmed within the human population. A large Swedish study in 1977 clearly demonstrated that abnormal deliveries are more common in zinc-deficient mothers, the major abnormality being either premature or post-mature labour. Unfortunately, this essential and somewhat simple antenatal information seems to have bypassed mainstream medicine. 'Foresight', the organization of preconceptual care, has made a number of very sensible recommendations about zinc and other mineral replacement, both preconceptually and during pregnancy.

Chromium

Schroeder, in his book *Trace Elements and Man* (published by Devlin Adair Publishing Company, Connecticut), makes a strong case for implicating chromium deficiency in the development of arterial disease. It seems that both arterial disease and diabetes can be correlated with low chromium levels in tissues (hair) and blood (serum). Our diets in general are chromium deficient, and chromium is not efficiently absorbed from either the small or large intestine. However, if enormous doses of chromium are given orally, then some does seem to get through into the tissues.

In our experience a large percentage of patients with diabetes have low chromium levels. If enormous oral doses of chromium are given, this seems to correct the tissue imbalance and make the diabetes far more responsive to simple treatment; for instance, insulin requirements decrease dramatically and the diabetes seems to become much 'milder'.

Malabsorption

Malabsorption really means the failure to absorb food and chemicals properly. In many food sensitivities the lining of the gastro-intestinal tract is disturbed so that absorption of many chemicals is abnormal. Some authorities have suggested that large and partially digested molecules are absorbed by the gut in this abnormal state, making food sensitivity more likely. Patients with multiple food sensitivities often demonstrate a generalized 'malabsorption' on hair analysis. This means that nearly all the minerals and vitamins are low and it is difficult to pinpoint any specific deficiencies. Occasionally there may be heavy metal poisoning with lead, but this is not a normal accompaniment. In

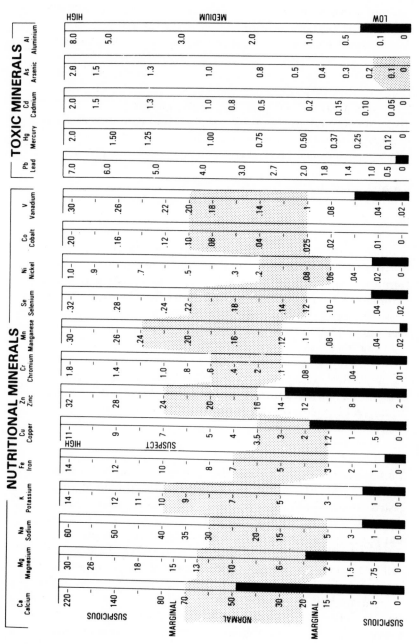

Figure 10: Hair analysis showing malabsorption.

such instances broad spectrum vitamin and mineral replacement should be carried out, and high doses should be used, combined with appropriate food exclusion.

Conclusion

Hair analysis is an important, simple, painless and relatively cheap method of looking at the state of health or disease of body tissues. Gross abnormalities in the trace metals may underpin the development of multiple food and chemical sensitivities; in other words, they may act as a trigger and can in fact be the fundamental cause of development of an ecological problem. If simple food exclusion does not seem to be an adequate method of managing a problem, then hair analysis is an important and useful investigation.

Addresses where hair analysis can be obtained

Trace Analysis Laboratory, P.O. Box 4235, Hayward, California 94540.

Foresight, The Old Vicarage, Church Lane, Witley, Godalming, Surrey, GU8 5PN.

Larkhall Laboratories, 225 Putney Bridge Road, London SW15 2PY.

11. Candida Sensitivity (Thrush)

As an ecologist, one is often faced by the question, 'What precipitated these sensitivities?' or, 'How did my allergies begin?'. In many instances a clear history of food sensitivity can be traced back to the patient's childhood, with episodes of colic and recurrent urinary tract infections occurring frequently in their early years. But many problems, particularly in women, present with no obvious ecological history.

The Pill

Dr Ellen Grant, previously at the migraine clinic in London, has suggested one possible reason to explain this phenomenon. Many women in the United Kingdom are taking artificial female hormones, in the oral contraceptive pill. We are well aware that the oral contraceptive has been of enormous value as a birth-control device and has also been one of the most important methods by which women have been liberated from the drudgery of perpetual pregnancy. However, such benefits have to be paid for and one of the costs has involved a clear increase in ecological problems among those taking the pill.

Dr Grant has argued that many of the known metabolic abnormalities produced by the pill (these include decrease in tissue zinc, an increase in tissue copper, altered liver function, alterations in a wide variety of hormonal levels and gross changes in the function of many enzymes) could predispose a prospective mother to produce malformed children. Studies have been published suggesting that those people taking oral contraceptives do have an increased rate of miscarriage and that many of the aborted foetuses are in fact abnormal. One of the major reasons for women stopping the oral contraceptive pill is multiple vague symptomatology such as headache, anxiety, weight gain, mood changes and irregular vaginal bleeding. All these symptoms seem in our view to correspond very closely with the sort of undifferentiated illness that frequently occurs in clinical ecology. Many of these effects are aggravated by smoking, but even without tobacco a growing body of hard evidence is emerging that suggests that in a small group of women the pill can and does precipitate illness. Consequently one of the answers to the question of why an ecological problem develops may well be the contraceptive pill.

Thrush

One of the more common complaints associated with the pill is recurrent thrush. The pill alters and depresses the immune system and changes the acidity of vaginal secretions. Both these effects predispose to infection, and thrush is the most common result.

Thrush is caused by a fungus, Candida albicans, which is a yeast that is found on all normal skin. In a healthy person there is a good balance between a multitude of different and harmless bacteria on the skin, in the mouth, bowel and vagina. Each bacteria (or fungus) secretes various chemicals which keep the growth of the others in check. A sort of natural balance is established, which if left undisturbed promotes normal wound healing and stops other more harmful bacteria causing dangerous infections. If there is a slight change in this normal environment, organisms such as Candida can multiply uncontrollably, resulting in local inflammation and irritation of the tissue. The Candida often lodges deep in tissues, for instance in the vagina; it invades not just the one or two surface cells but penetrates deep into the lining of the external tissue. The major symptoms produced are soreness and a white discharge. Acute infection or overgrowth of Candida (acute Candidiasis or thrush) can occur in young children, particularly in the mouth or gastro-intestinal tract, in the urinary system of both males and females, and in adult males it may present as a sore penis (balanitis).

There are a number of factors that predispose to thrush as well as the oral contraceptive pill. If a deficient immune state exists, such as in a patient with cancer or one who is receiving large doses of steroids (hydrocortisone), then infection with Candida is more likely. Young babies with immature immune systems (particularly breast-fed babies) are at risk, as are the old and infirm. Antibiotics are one of the most commonly used drugs in the West. These chemicals kill off harmful *and* healthy bacteria, predisposing to an overgrowth of organisms such as Candida which may in turn cause thrush.

In most people the odd, acute attack of vaginal or oral thrush is harmless and with adequate conventional treatment and a normal immune system, the problem will resolve completely. The normal therapy given is an antifungal agent such as Nystatin. However, in a few people the Candidiasis keeps occurring and is almost impossible to treat. This chronic or recurrent acute infection can cause immeasurable problems.

Chronic thrush

If a fungus lodges in the deep tissues of any structure, it will be almost impossible to dislodge permanently with conventional antifungals. It seems as if these drugs just suppress the symptoms and as soon as they are stopped further symptomatology reoccurs. Candida is a very allergenic organism and highly adept at triggering the body's immune system into activity. The symptoms attributable to chronic Candidiasis (by ecologists) are almost endless, and vary from vaginal irritation to malaise and headache. The first ecologist to recognise this problem was an American, Dr Orion Truss.

Patients with multiple food sensitivities

A small but distinct group of patients have multiple and variable food sensitivities. Patients with rheumatoid arthritis may respond well to an exclusion diet of wheat, oats, rye, potatoes and tomatoes for about five or six weeks and then suddenly relapse for no apparent reason. A sensitivity to milk, and sickness, may then develop and again a short-term response occurs followed by a relapse. Perhaps somebody with inhaled sensitivities may keep changing the end points of their desensitizing solutions, such fluctuations occurring almost weekly.

These problems are very difficult to control and almost always signify an underlying abnormality that if not treated will make an ecological approach to the problem of limited value. In some instances the underlying abnormality might be heavy metal poisoning (as discussed in Chapter 10), but in others chronic Candidiasis could well be the problem.

In other words a simple and common event like the prescription of the contraceptive pill predisposes to thrush and, in a small group of women, the consequent development of chronic Candidiasis. This in turn unbalances the body so that multiple and fluctuant ecological problems develop and continue until the Candida is completely removed from the system. Sensitivity to Candida can be diagnosed by a variety of investigations, including intradermal injection testing.

Treatment
As we have already mentioned, chronic Candidiasis cannot be adequately treated with conventional therapy. In our experience it will only suppress symptoms and either acute Candidiasis or other chronic symptomatology will develop after therapy has been stopped. Chronic Candidiasis can *only* be abolished by using minimal dose therapy. Either by dilution of Candida using the Miller technique, or by using homoeopathic doses of Candida — such as Candida 30c, one tablet every morning; or Candida 200c, one tablet once a week. Such therapy will almost always allow other subsequent food sensitivities to settle and the whole unbalanced situation will usually resolve over a period of therapy lasting for at least three and possibly nine months.

Chronic Candidiasis, like heavy metal poisoning, can underlie food sensitivity. If such underlying factors are present, then the patient with food or chemical sensitivity is unlikely to gain symptomatic improvement on a diet or with desensitization if the primary event is left undiagnosed and untreated.

12. Epilogue

Where do we go from here?
This book has suggested a number of controversial ideas, and they contain the seeds of the next steps forward. Before these steps can be taken effectively a lot of groundwork remains to be done.

Increased recognition of ecological illness
The existence of ecological illness needs to be more widely recognized by doctors and patients alike. It is still a minority approach to illness by doctors and by many it is regarded as cranky. Convincing evidence is steadily accumulating that many patients are ill because of their environment. There is little evidence, however, that the publication of learned papers influences the way doctors practise. Changing medical fashion is probably the biggest factor in affecting the way medicine is practised, much to the continued embarrassment of the bastions of academic medicine. Hopefully this book will be a step in the right direction, as we have tried to be critical of both the conventional and ecological approach and therefore we feel we have presented a balanced view.

Education of doctors
Doctors receive no training in the management of ecological illness. Those that have an interest have usually picked up their expertise from patients, and through various books often written for the lay public. A few have attended one of the rare training courses available in ecology. Many doctors with such an interest often suffer

from ecologically based illnesses themselves. Our experience has been that there was nowhere for us to go to learn ecology — hardly a useful scenario for us to develop our skills. This situation has been remedied to a limited extent, and our Centre devotes some of its time to training doctors in ecology. One day medical students may learn it as undergraduates, but this is probably many years away.

Research

As must be apparent from this book, ecology is full of unexplained findings, indicating an obvious need for more research. In terms of research funding, ecology has been a Cinderella but there are signs that things are changing. Research is needed on two fronts, clinical trials and basic mechanisms. The major lack is research into basic mechanisms of sensitivity, as it is only when we understand these better that we can usefully modify treatment programmes. More innovative work is needed, as conventional explanations of allergy break down when applied to ecology.

Holism

Holism seems to be the up and coming fashion, and has come to mean the recognition and treatment of all aspects of the patient's problem. We believe that this is a major step forward, as it encourages a broad view of illness and discourages a narrow specialist approach. The specialist approach still dominates, but things are changing. Ecologists themselves have often been guilty of a narrow approach, and they will have to stand back and recognize the existence of underlying conditions in ecological illness. Only when a holistic approach, as exemplified in general practice, carries the same sort of respect given to specialist medicine, can these new approaches be researched in an unprejudiced manner.

Changes in the patient's environment

So far all the steps forward have largely been directed at doctors; but what about the patient? People are now more ecologically aware, as it becomes generally accepted that we live on a planet with finite resources. The fact of pollution is universally recognized and encouraging steps are being taken to improve our environment.

These ideas are beginning to find political expression, albeit in embryonic form at the time of writing, in the German Green Party and the British Ecology Party. It is likely that these innovative political movements will become of major importance over the next half-century.

On a personal level, everyone would be wise to limit ecologically dangerous exposure. The use of aerosol sprays, garden pesticides and weedkillers and artificial fertilizers should be stopped. The wise man will grow the majority of his own food requirements and collect and drink rain water. Drug exposure should be kept to a minimum and processed foods of all sorts should be avoided. All these measures will lead to a more healthy and fulfilling life.

Multi-national and governmental action

Perhaps the most important changes have to be brought about by multi-national companies and governments. Ironically, multi-nationals often appear to wield more power than governments, but so long as their decisions are based purely on economic considerations, then we can't hope to move much further forward. Ecological awareness doesn't make profits, but it enables us all to live a more healthy and fulfilled life. There are signs that multi-nationals will respond to public pressure, but much still remains to be done.

Governments will hopefully continue to pass anti-pollution legislation, such as banning lead in petrol. As a result of public campaigning it now appears at least possible that lead will be banned from petrol in the United Kingdom within the foreseeable future, in spite of opposition from the oil and car industries. Many other well-directed, vigorous and hard-hitting public campaigns are needed, as this is how change is brought about — the anti-nuclear campaign is a good example. We hope that this book will encourage those many people who are trying to change things, but appear to be losing all the time, that success will come if only they persist.

In conclusion we have tried to present a balanced view of ecology, indicating areas where it ought to change. We have also given as much advice as has been possible in a book of this size. We haven't made it a book of diets or of food lists. Such books are readily available and are listed under Further Reading at the end of this book. We have tried to make people think and so we have been deliberately controversial — it seemed a waste of effort to write the same book on ecology that other people have written. The next few years will show us whether we have been successful or not.

Further Reading

Not All in the Mind by Richard Mackarness (Pan Paperbacks)
Chemical Victims by Richard Mackarness (Pan Paperbacks)

Both these books give a good general introduction to food and chemical sensitivity and are written for the lay public.

Allergies, Your Hidden Enemy by T. G. Randolph and Ralph Moss
   (Turnstone Press, Wellingborough, Northamptonshire)

This is a more detailed book written by American authors, but doesn't give any further ideas than the books by Richard Mackarness.

For doctors and other health professionals, the following books may be of interest:

Food Allergy by J. B. Miller (Charles C. Thomas, Illinois, USA)

This gives a detailed guide on desensitization techniques.

Food Allergy by Randolph Rinkel and Zeller (Charles C. Thomas,
   Illinois, USA)
Clinical Ecology by L. D. Dickey (Charles C. Thomas, Illinois, USA)
Introduction to Clinical Allergy by B. F. Feingold (Charles C.
   Thomas, Illinois, USA)
Why Your Child Is Hyperactive by B. F. Feingold (Random House
   Press, New York)

All of these books can be regarded as textbooks of clinical ecology;

they are all American books and suffer, like many medical textbooks from America, in that they could all be condensed to a quarter of the size without losing any informational content.

For those interested in a critical scientific review of ecology from the orthodox medical point of view, the following book will be of interest:

Food Intolerance and Food Aversion. A joint report of the Royal College of Physicians and the British Nutrition Foundation. Reprinted from the Royal College of Physicians of London, Vol. 18, No. 2, April 1984. This excellent report provides considerable support from conventional doctors for the use of food avoidance as a treatment for many complaints.

Clinical Reactions to Food edited by M. H. Lessof (John Wiley and Sons, Chichester, West Sussex)

For those interested in the electrical techniques for testing and diagnosing underlying disorders and also ACR testing, the following books may be of interest:

Modern Techniques of Acupuncture, Volume I and II, by Julian Kenyon (Thorsons Publishers, Wellingborough, Northamptonshire)

Short Manual of the Vegatest Method by Helmut Schimmel, edited by Julian Kenyon (Vega Griesshaber GmbH, 7622 Schiltach, Schwalzwald, West Germany)

The Segmental Electrogram by Helmut Schimmel, edited by Julian Kenyon (Vega Griesshaber GmbH, 7622 Schiltach, Schwalzwald, West Germany)

For those interested in the work done on monitoring electromagnetic change around the body in order to elucidate the mechanism of food and chemical sensitivity, the following book may be of interest:

Electrographic Imaging in Medicine and Biology by Ion Dimitrescu, edited by Julian Kenyon (Neville Spearman, Sudbury, Suffolk)

Index